CW00614032

Above the Void

By Nick Hooper

To Judith
my love

Nick xxx

Self-Published by Wordandnote Publishing 2017

www.wordandnote.com

Copyright Nick Hooper 2017

ISBN 978-1-9997848-0-5

A CIP catalogue reference for this book
is available from the British Library.

This book is a work of fiction. Names, characters, businesses, organizations, places and events are either the product of the author's imagination or are used fictitiously. Any resemblance to actual persons, living or dead, events or locations is entirely coincidental.

Typeset by Lucy Ayrton

Printed and bound in Great Briton by 4edge Limited

Cover design by Tony Davis

Dedicated to my mum, Muriel Hooper, who taught me to write when I was ten, and introduced me to so many great books, including her own, which have influenced so much of my writing.

Observations

Privileged Information. 07.23.2014
US E3-Sentry early-warning aircraft reported sighting small black fast-moving flying object at 29000 feet. Craft placed on alert as they tracked the unidentified object. It was identified as a raven appearing to be flying at impossibly high speed. Captain reported having sighted whooper swans at this altitude in the past, but never a raven.

South of Nuuk, Bird Observation field station Greenland. 07.23.2014
Raven observed flying low over our field station in an eastward direction, apparently gliding effortlessly at high speed against the westward wind current. Noted down as unusual sighting.

Sermilik, Greenland. 07.23.2014
Raven observed flying low over Sermilik field station apparently having no trouble making good headway against prevailing wind. Speed very fast - impossible to estimate. Noted down as unusual sighting. Nuuk have a similar report, but it couldn't possibly be the same bird.

The Accident

Chapter 1

Melissa stood just a bit too close to the edge of the cliff. She could hear the distant thump of the waves meeting the shingle beach far below. The sea spread out before her, a moving counterpane, and she felt it would be so tempting at that moment to jump off the edge and glide the two hundred feet down into its gentle swell – glinting grey, blue and green as the morning sunlight caught it. She could smell the salty damp of it – it filled her with its freshness.

Behind her was her old life – the farmhouse, drab and half empty, his things gone. They had hardly exchanged a word. Their love was like dead flowers: blooms, petals, stamens all fallen off leaving the wrinkled browning stems in stagnant smelly water. She was left to clear up, clear out. A sad end to their life together. She wasn't bitter, she was numb – that was all. She couldn't feel... anything. No babies, no family, no job – nothing.

And yet, there was something. Something round the corner just out of reach – out of sight. She was a survivor. No jumping off the cliff. She could see it in her mind's eye.

'Melissa Jenkins found dead at bottom of cliff. Ex-husband said she was fine when he left her... deda, deda, dead'.

No she wouldn't jump, she would fly, or do the nearest thing to it. She turned round and walked back to the farmhouse, and looked at the pile of her belongings that she had stacked outside the front door. She carried the few cases and boxes to the fallen-down barn, picked up her bicycle, and cycled down the hill towards the village to find someone who would take her belongings to the station. The wind filled her hair. The feeling of speed and exhilaration filled her body as she pedalled faster and faster down the smooth single track road to the village tucked in right at the bottom of the valley. Sheltered, homely, and hopefully, helpful.

The sea was just to her left, the green fields and patchwork landscape to her right. No traffic on this lonely road. Only her. And her thoughts. But they were being blown away by the wind in her face – just her and her bike going downhill at speed.

Free.

Always before, she had cycled down that hill knowing she would have to pedal laboriously up it again to an increasingly uncertain welcome at the top. Hard, hard suffering. Sweat and pain, for what? But now she was flying down the hill never to return. She would find someone to fetch her belongings and she would be gone.

Down in the village the clock on the church tower showed it was just after twelve. Melissa got off her bike, and walked into the pub opposite.

"Half a pint of Wye, Bert, please, and do you know of anyone who could fetch my stuff from the farm and bring it to the station?" She was still out of breath when she came out with this stream of requests, as if it was urgent. But actually, she had plenty of time. She had nowhere to go. No train to catch.

Bert looked slightly startled. The normally laid-back hippy-girl, that had come to his pub regularly over the last couple of years, had sped up into a dusty racing demon with the wind in her hair and the sun glinting in her eyes.

"Sorry to hear about you and Mike," he stuttered clumsily. "I mean, you know…" He stumbled to a halt. A shadow of self-doubt crossed his face… and then it was gone. He smiled, "Have this on the house, I'll give Sam's Taxis a ring for you if you like. They'll take care of you. What time's your train?"

She hadn't thought that far. She didn't even really know where she would go. Mum's was… toxic. Dad had disappeared again. And Daniel? No she couldn't go back there.

"I don't know which one I'm catching yet," her truth concealing a lie. "But if someone can get my stuff to the station… I can sort it out."

Suddenly she felt a bit pathetic. Sort it out! Sort what out? She looked round the pub. It was nearly empty. The lunchtime drinkers hadn't appeared yet and only a couple of walkers were there, hunched over a table looking at their map. Oh, and in the corner there was Leery O'Leary. What was he looking at her like that for? Creep. With his drinker's paunch and his roaming hands. And those teeth. She shivered involuntarily. No, she wouldn't go over there. Stay at the bar and sip her beer. Just try to remember it wasn't a glass of water.

Bert followed her gaze. "He's been spending most of his time here since he lost his wife." He said quietly, "He's harmless enough poor sod. Just drinking for Ireland. Used to be a good singer, probably still would be if he could remember the words." He paused, and then realised what he was meant to be doing. "I'll just go and phone them now."

Well, that will teach me to be so prejudiced, she thought, he's a fellow traveller. Curious how life brought you the unexpected. She shifted her gaze to the half open door, the sun shining in from the street and lighting up the dancing particles of dust, never settling, always on the move. She used to think of them as fairies when she was little, and now she just gazed at them, allowing her mind to switch off - thinking back through her life in a dreamlike way to how she had got here. It didn't look so bad to start with, looking at it like that. Not such a tragedy.

A blessed childhood.

At least until the happening. But she wouldn't go there, not now.

Her mind went back to the rambling old mansion where she was brought up. Bits had been added on through the centuries, and by the time you got to the front of the building you'd time-travelled five hundred years to the eighteenth century, with its ornate plaster ceilings. Set in an acre of garden, this crumbling house provided a leaky and sometimes chilly residence for three families of humans and at least ten families of mice. The mice were kept in check by traps, poison, frying pans and anything else the humans could lay their hands on. But the humans increased in number in a most prolific manner – all three families boasting a large number of children sprawling through attics and cellars, kitchens and hallways.

Her own family lived on the ground floor, occupying the lower regions. Her mother's cousin's family had the first floor, and all the grandeur that went with it, and her father's sister Doris was up on the top floor with her smoker husband tch, tch, and their numerous boys. Auntie Doris was her favourite grown-up in time of need. Always had time for her. Always had a bicky and a drink, a listening ear, and a soft word. A refuge. Even with all those boys: Denis, Dan, Darren, Damian etc., she could still get her place with their mum. They were always off doing something in one of the small rooms that led off the attic that the boys all slept in. One massive room, she remembered - beds laid out like a dorm. But that was where the likeness to school ended. They all had freedom. A lot of freedom.

Maybe too much...

Things were a bit stiffer and more formal on the first floor. Good behaviour was expected, and there were the ornaments. Ornaments everywhere. On shelves, on tables, in the little alcoves that were so great to hide in. The potential for breakage was massive. And these ornaments were dusted every day. Mum's cousin Iris thought that children should be seen and not heard. How she managed to live a floor away from Doris and co., Melissa never understood. Being the youngest of the whole tribe, there was a lot she didn't understand at the time. A lot.

"He said he'd pick them up this afternoon about two. Is that OK? Or do you want to speak to him love?" Bert's voice jolted her out of her reverie. The motes of dust were still flying about in the sunshine, and she looked down at her glass. Empty. How did that happen?

"Oh, er, thanks, that sounds good." What was she talking about? What sounds good? She didn't know where she was going, or even when.

The pub was beginning to fill up. Early lunchtime drinkers were filtering in, getting their pints and sitting in their accustomed corners. And there she was with an empty glass. Not half full, not half empty. Just empty.

She managed to catch Bert's attention after he had served a particularly large member of the lunchtime fraternity, so tall and wide that he seemed to blot out the sun and the rest of the bar for a moment.

"Another half of Wye please Bert," she said half apologetically. If she carried on drinking at this rate, she'd never make it out of the pub and into her future - whatever that was going to be. She never drank much: two halves in an evening. Alcohol had a very strong effect on her. She didn't get maudlin or aggressive - just talkative and friendly. But now she was drinking without feeling much at all. She'd better talk to someone or leave. No possibility of that - most of the men, and they were all men, were either huddled together talking to each other or looking like they didn't want to talk to anyone.

But there was Leery O'Leary. Sitting in the corner on his own, looking round the pub with his soggy old eyes, hoping someone would talk to him. She went over to his table and sat down. He looked her over in that creepy way he had, and she shuddered but swallowed hard and tried to concentrate on the fact that he was a human being.

"All alone love?" he asked. "No one with you today?"

"No, just me." She tried furiously to think of something to say. "Er, lovely day isn't it." The sun, shining through the grimy

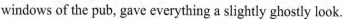

windows of the pub, gave everything a slightly ghostly look.

"Is it? Oh all days are the same to me, love." He wasn't going to help get this conversation off the ground, so she took a big swig of her beer and tried again.

"Um, I'm just moving out – leaving the farm…"

"Sounds good sense to me," said Leery. "Wish I'd moved away when I had the chance, but I've got my council flat now and there's nowhere else to go."

"Yes, well, I'm going… somewhere. Not quite sure where yet." She looked down into her glass. That second half pint had almost disappeared, and her head was beginning to swim.

"You should go off travelling. Young girl like you. Take your opportunities while you can. That's what I say." He gazed round the room as if searching for someone else to talk to.

Abruptly, he turned and looked straight into her eyes. His sad dog-like expression had gone , and was replaced by a piercing look – shrewd and bitter.

"Go! Leave! Get out of here girl, while you have the chance. This is no place for you. You don't belong here." He said this under his breath and then looked away.

She felt fear then. Fear of no future – no place to go. Her heavy tear-laden past dragging her down with clammy fingers. She wanted to get out, out into the fresh air and sunlight, before all her optimism was sucked out of her. She scrambled to her feet knocking over the chair, and ran out of the pub, and straight into the road.

There was a squeal of tyres, she felt a huge force push her off her feet, a deadening blow to the back of her head, and everything stopped.

Hospital

Chapter 2

"Can you smell that funny smell?" It's my mum's voice. "Smells like burning rubber." I'm surrounded by smoke, and there's shouting. "Get out! Get out now! No, don't get your dolly. Get out Melissa... Melissa... Melissa..." The desperate voices change gradually into someone calling me gently just by my ear.

Slowly a ceiling comes into focus – white, stark with painfully bright lights set into it. Mechanical and cold, it bears down on me till it seems like my head will burst. That's it, my head's going to explode. Somewhere there is deep, deep pain trying to get out. I try to turn my head to see who's been calling my name, but I can't. Something's holding my head firmly in place. I try to say, "What am I doing here?" But the effort involved in moving my mouth is too great.

"Melissa? Nurse, she's come round." It's a man's voice.

I can hear movement: footsteps, a clattering, and suddenly a disembodied face appears looking down at me, then another. Male, female, I can't tell. Just pink shadows against the light.

They're all talking at once.

"Check..."

"Get the..."

"Call Doctor..."

More footsteps. More clattering. There's a piercing light in my eyes. I close them.

"Melissa? Can you hear me?" It's another man's voice – too loud.

I want them to go away. I want to be back in my old home, safe with my family. Was that a dream? Is this a dream? There's something horribly sharp and clinical here that tells me that this is reality. This is what I've come back to.

"She's conscious, but she can't move or speak... injury to the

11

back of … head …. cerebellum." Loud voice.

'Hello, I'm here,' I try to say. You wish you weren't. And what's a… a… cerebublium?

I'm so frustrated, I don't know why… I move something. Not sure what it is.

"Doctor, she moved her hand."

My hand.

"Hello, Melissa. Can you hear me?" That loud voice nagging at me again. "Move your hand if you can."

I try doing the same thing again, but the effort makes the ceiling start to descend again. They are all saying something – I can't make out what it is because they're getting quieter and everything's fading… out.

In.

It feels like I'm in the middle of a snowstorm, inside a tiny glass dome. I can't make sense of anything. I feel numb but inside me there's a deep, deep pain... somewhere.

Won't go away, go away, go away…

Out.

In.

"Tell June I've got a…"

"If you'll just listen. He's got to go to…"

I catch conversations from somewhere. Not for me, but I can't block them out. I panic: will I be stuck with these conversations for ever…for ever…for ever..?

Out.

In.

More pain. More numbness. I've got this storm going on in my head. I must get to the centre. I must find…something. There're beeps too – outside me. Beep, beep... Can I control these beeps?

Are they part of me? Then the clatter... then...

Out.

In.

I'm awake again.

No-one is here.

I feel something. Something familiar. Something I shouldn't do. I'm peeing in my bed. I mustn't pee in my bed, but I can't stop myself. But there's no warm wet feeling. Pee just gone...

gone...

Out.

In.

Beep, beep, beep...

Is this part of me?

I start to panic: the beeps get faster. Oh no, it is me. Can I do anything?

"Doctor. I think she needs more se...da...tive..."

The numbness increases.

The beeps get slower... fade

out...

In.

The storm's not so bad now. I think I'm upside down, but at least things are stiller. White light in my eyes. "Leave me alone," I say. "Don't you understand? I CAN'T stand... you. Go away, go away..."

Out.

In.

I'm lying on a bed of warm seaweed.

Everything's calmed down.

The snowstorm, was it a snowstorm? It's gone.

Still, still light.
I'm looking up.
A face appears.
I want that face.
I love that face.
It goes away.
No!
Beep, beep, beep. Speeds up – slows down – fades
out.

Chapter 3

I am running down a smoke-filled hall. There are cries all around me. Children screaming, "Mummy, Daddy!" Parents calling – their voices full of panic. Everybody's running. The ceiling above me groans and shrieks – it is coming down. I look up and it starts to glow white. It must be the heat.

But as I look it stops and stays just where it is hovering above me - caught in suspended animation.

"I'm so sorry." The voice is gentle. "You ran out straight in front of me." He is talking quietly by my left ear, at least I think it's left. "Why did you do it? Why did you run out like that?" I love this man's voice – it takes my mind away from the nightmare.

"I asked in the pub later, but no-one knew why you'd run out like that. Apparently you'd been talking to an old drunk in the corner, but when I asked him, he didn't say anything. Just stared at me as if I was mad."

He's just talking to himself – he doesn't know I'm awake. Maybe he's mad, but he doesn't sound mad. I'm not mad either – I'm making sense of this. This is about me. What I did. Once.

"The landlord was great. He stayed with me while we waited for the ambulance. He said you'd just split up with your husband. He said he'd arranged for your things to be taken to the station. I wonder where you were going."

I wonder that too. Husband? Can't remember. Hurts to try. Too far away.

"You are a complete mystery. You don't seem to have anyone. The hospital tried contacting your family, and finally found your mother. She came to visit you. Brought some cheap flowers. They're dead already. But she didn't seem to care. Not really. Just talked about herself. She says she'll come back."

My mother? Who is she? Do I want her?

He pauses. Then I feel something. It's my hand - he's taken hold of my hand. I feel something rush through me: fear, love, desire.

"I'm here though. I come when I'm not working. I like talking to you. You remind me of someone." There's something moving about the way he says that, and I want to give his hand a squeeze. He lets go and his face appears above me. I see him clearly for the first time. Gentle boyish face, a bit like a choirboy.

I saw him before. I'm sure I saw him before. I remember the love I felt. I want to reach up and touch his cheek, but there's no chance of that. I can't fucking move my fucking arm.

He looks into my eyes. I blink.

"Nurse, she's come round again."

"I'll call Doctor Sharma. Doctor Napier's off today."

His face goes away again, but I hear him by me. Close to my head.

"I'm James." His voice sounds urgent. "I... Alice... She died in a car accident."

Go away Malice, I want to say.

"It was a couple of years ago now. But it's so strange that I should have... that this should have happened now. That's what I wanted to tell you, so you didn't think I was some kind of weirdo."

Deirdre weirdo, malice Alice? Who's she?

"Mr Penhaligon, we need to see Melissa now." A gentle female Indian voice interrupts us, and I hear him get up.

"See you in a bit." Says Mister Pen-a-lot-again.

No, no, come back.

I hear the sound of curtains being pulled. Curtains – my shroud. There's some bustling about and something rattling by my bed.

A woman leans over me and looks into my eyes. She must be quite short as her face is much closer to mine than that lovely man's was. Her dark brown complexion and curved nose, pierced with a tiny diamond make me feel like I'm in Indi... Indi...I can't remember the name.

She smiles. "Hello. I'm going to shine a light into your eyes. Please try to keep them open for me."

The light is blinding. Painful. I want to close my eyes, but keep them open as best I can. I like her. I want to please her.

"Good, good. Thank you. Can you talk?"

I could try. I send the message 'yes' to my mouth. I feel it move – it takes a massive effort, I'm sure I said yes. But the woman goes away. There's a murmur of voices, but nothing distinct. Except one word.

"Cerebellum."

Cerebublium? Did I hear that word earlier? I'm not sure. Have I got one? Is that the problem?

There's the sound of those curtains again. Some shuffling, and then whispered, "You can have ten minutes, and then we must give her her medication." A female voice I don't recognise. Sharp. Bossy. Ugh.

A scraping sound, and then I feel warm breath on my cheek.

"Hello. It's James again. I guess you can't talk, but you're awake. That's such good news. I've come every day, waiting for you to wake up."

I want to turn my head and look at him. I try to move, but suddenly, the deep pain that's been hovering round the edge of my consciousness, comes into focus, and I get a message that says 'DON'T DO THAT.'

"I have been able to come and see you every day because of my work. I work mainly at home but partly in this hospital. At home I work as a psychotherapist, and then I run a cancer counselling clinic here in the hospital."

Cancer? I don't have cancer do I? I remember that cancer was something horrible and I feel a cold shiver go down my body. Is the cere-wotsit-um something to do with that?

"That finishes at five, so I can come and see you then. Sometimes earlier if something changes. I suspect they'll cut the clinic soon. Everything's being cut. But I'm fortunate enough to have my own private work."

He pauses, and I wonder why he's telling me all this. Does he love me?

"I don't know why I'm telling you all this. You're not my patient, but I do know that company is healing when you're recovering from a serious injury. When I knocked you down..."

His voice goes a bit gravelly.

I love him. I love him so much. Oh no. I want to pee.

"When I knocked you down, you hit the back of your head on the road." He clears his throat. "The blow damaged the nerve routes to your cerebellum."

I can't stop myself. I'll wet my bed. Someone will tell me off. But I can't feel the wet, and what's this thing that keeps coming up? Cere... cere...

"The part of your brain that controls movement and speech. This is why it's so hard for you to talk. You can't move anyway. They've put your head and shoulders in a brace to protect things while they mend."

So things are going to mend? How long will I be stuck here like this? How long have I been stuck like this? My mind whizzes backwards and forwards. I'm losing my grip.

"There'll be therapies to help you get things working again, but for now they say you must rest. And here I am, helping you rest... I hope."

He really doesn't sound like a, like a... wots-ellor. He's so eager to please me. He loves me, that's it he loves me, and I love him. I love him so.

"I can see Matron coming. She'll be giving you your medication."

I hear an edge to his voice. Doesn't he like Megatron?

"Mr Penhaligon. I'll have to…"

"It's alright, I'm off now." He puts his hand on mine, and for a moment as he leans forward, I catch a glimpse of his expression, and I see a vulnerability. He is not god-like at that moment – he's a boy. Don't go lovely boy. Don't go and leave me with this harsh, edgy-voiced Megatron. As I start to cry, I feel a surge of something cool going into my system, and I don't want to be in this any more.

So I'm out.

Chapter 4

I am so cold. It's so dark. I'm caught in a snowdrift and can't get out because there's somebody holding onto my leg. I pull and pull and at last I am free. But too late – I haven't the energy to carry on. I just lie back in the snow and look up at the sun. It's so bright that I want to look away but I can't. I can't move my head. I can't move anything. The bright light bears down on me, but it's not the sun. I'm in that house with the smoke and fire, and the ceiling's coming down.

"Sorry love. My hands are cold. They're always cold."

A woman talking to herself.

"There."

The ceiling comes into focus. It's not going to crush me. It's that hospital ceiling again and I'm back in hospital. How long has it been? How long will it go on – this to and fro from dreaming to waking? It occurs to me that she doesn't know I'm awake.

"Hello," I say in my head, but what I hear is scarcely audible.

I try again. "Hello." That was louder, it took all my strength. Anyway, she's heard me. Her face appears – the gentle lines of a woman in her fifties. She smiles.

"Hello love. Are you awake? Did you say something?"

I blink.

"Good. I'll call Doctor Ford. She said to let her know if you came round."

Doctor Ward on her ward round. I wonder if it will be called Ward's ward. Perhaps she'll get an award for warding off disease on her Ward ward. Hello, my mind's pattering on again. But at least it's working. I'm warm now under my sheets and blankets. I luxuriate in this feeling of bed-ness. I wriggle my toes. I WRIGGLE MY TOES!

Nurse is coming back with Doctor Ward. I hear the clatter of their sensible shoes on the ward floor.

Doctor Ward's broad pleasant face appears above me.

Doctor Ward wears makeup. I'm surprised she has time to put it on, what with all the work she must do on her ward. She looks into my eyes.

"Hello, I'm Doctor Ford," says a fruity friendly voice. "How are we?"

I don't know how well you are Doctor, but I feel much better thank you. AND I can wriggle my toes!

"Very well," I say, but it sounds like 'eh-i-eh', and it's so quiet.

"Hello, can you hear me?" She looks closer into my eyes.

I blink.

Doctor Ward-ward goes off-camera. "I think we should get Doctor Park the neurologist. Can you find him, Nurse? He'll be in his consulting room. Fourth floor."

Clatter of nurse's feet off into the distance. I follow the sound and hear voices: "No June, I don't want you to do that. He's…"

"Now, let's take a look at you." Doctor Ward-ward grunts as she bends down. I feel her breath on my ear. Another grunt as she straightens up and clatters round the end of my bed. I wriggle my toes as she goes past, but she can't see them under the sheets of course. I guess she's looking at instruments and things that must be attached to me by wires and tubes.

Wires and tubes, wires and tubes.

"All looking tickety-boo."

Her face appears again. "We'll have to find a way of communicating with you. Mark will know. Still, you're mending well."

But I did just try and communicate. She just didn't hear me.

There's the sound of footsteps – soft shoes this time.

"Ah, James. Do you want to keep her company while we try and find Doctor Park? I've got some more visits to do. She's looking better."

22

And I can wriggle my toes.

A handsome boyish face looks down at me. He's the one I love, isn't he?

"Hello," I say.

"Doctor, she said something." He disappears for a moment.

"Oh too late. Pat's always on the move." His face reappears, and he smiles.

"I'm really pleased to see you looking so much better today."

Today? So I've been out since yesterday. What happened in-between?

"When Mark comes we'll find a way to communicate with you. We don't know quite how you've been affected by the... by the accident. I think you're doing fine, but..." His voice trails off, and his face disappears. There's the scrape of a chair being pulled up.

"I hope you don't mind me talking to you like this. It's supposed to do you good, and it's good for me too. I might be a therapist and a counsellor, but right now I'm the man who knocked you down, and I want you to get better." His voice has gone all gravelly – that's because he loves me, of course.

"I've been doing some cancer counselling today. There're some brave people there..." He's cheering up now. "Tonight I'll go home to my house and light a fire in the sitting room. I like my house – it has good memories, and I enjoy a good glass of red wine in front of the fire."

Do I drink wine? No I don't drink wine. I don't drink anything. Bad for me.

"It's a little Victorian coal fire. The house was built in the twenties, but I got the fireplace from a junkyard and fitted it. It makes it all seem much older, which I like. I only have one glass. Margaret River. I was there a few years ago with..." He gets stuck for a moment.

Margaret River, Margaret River, wasn't I there too? Was I with

23

him?

"I was there with Alice. Before… before the accident."

Is that my accident? Something stirs in my memory. Oh yes, someone died... For some reason it makes me feel uneasy. I dismiss it. I have other worries now. For instance, how can I get James to look at me wriggling my toes? How can I talk to him at all?

"Ah ooh er…er?" That was meant to be 'are you alright?' and it comes out as a whisper. Not even sure it is audible against the hum and clatter of Ward's ward.

"I thought of you last night." His voice brightens up again. "I imagined you as a child, in this big old rambling house, playing with your dolly. Silly I know… every girl must have a dolly at some stage… but the image of your house seemed so real as I looked into the fire."

Oh-my-God. The fire. There was a fire.

"There's so little I actually know about you. All the lines have dried up. Your mother…" His voice becomes harsh.

"But you will be able to tell me about yourself… soon." He pauses. I want to reach out to him – I love him so much. Hold his hand. I feel a movement. Was that my hand that moved?

His face appears above me. He looks puzzled. "You moved your hand. Are you trying to tell me something?" He smiles. "You are, aren't you!"

His hand touches mine. The hand I moved. I can feel the connection with him now. It goes up my arm, my shoulder, and spreads inside me, as though the warmth of his hand pulls the disconnected parts of my body together.

We stay like that for a long time. Then he sighs, and I hear the edgy voice of Megatron and I roll out of this world and into sleep.

Chapter 5

"Leave your dolly. We can't get that now." Mummy's shouting
now. *"James, James where are you?"* There are shrieks and
groans all around me, as the ceiling descends. I'm screaming.
Daddy's lost in the fire. The smoke is choking me. There are
voices everywhere, shouting, calling. I run in the confusion and
the ceiling starts coming down on me. It's so bright.

Too bright. These lights are too bright. And everyone's talking
at once.

"She shouldn't…"

"…a week since…"

"We must get things moving…"

"Needs rest…"

I try to shout, "Hello, I'm here." But it comes out as a moan:
'a-oh-ee-ere'.

Still, it has the desired effect. The voices stop, and a new face
appears in my field of vision. Dark, thinning hair. A face that
somehow reminds me of a lion.

"Hello. How are you feeling?" He has a deep voice like a lion.
Makes me think of Sean… Sean… can't remember his other
name.

How am I feeling? Er… headache's much better. But otherwise
the same. Can't move. Can't talk. Actually, not quite true. I can
move, yes, I can move both hands and my toes. It's not like I'm
paralysed, it just takes a huge effort. And speaking's the same. If
I shout it comes out as a whisper – a parody of what I am trying
to say.

"Frustrated!" I shout. Too much effort – the headache's getting
worse, and it just sounds like I'm wheezing.

"We want to do some tests…" he says – his voice rumbles in
a gentle way.

"Too early…"

"Mark, she's too tired…"

I hear Megatron's voice, and the-man-I-love. That's James isn't it? But not James Bond.

"But she can move her hand, you said." Mister Rumble's voice remains low and gentle, despite the negative sounds coming from the other two.

I move my hand obligingly. I wave and point towards my toes, but it feels hard to do the pointing – like all my fingers move together. Everything's so stiff and uncooperative.

But Mister Rumble's picked up my movement.

"You're right, she can move her hand." He hums to himself as he moves down the bed and lifts the sheets off my feet. I obligingly wriggle my toes.

"Ah yes…Well done, that's good, very good. There's movement right down her body, see? This is good news."

My body. MY body. Hello. It's me you're talking about.

"We could do another scan, but it's a bit early yet. I'm not sure we'd see much change." He growls gently to himself.

"Mark, she's listening to all this." The-man-I-love's voice intercedes on my behalf.

"Sorry." Mister Rumble's face appears again. "Sorry, I was getting carried away…"

Yes, you forgot I was here.

"… it all looks very good. You are able to move some muscles now, which is good news. The pathways to your cerebellum have been damaged in the accident, but they can repair themselves. At the moment you must feel that it's very hard to move anything at all. But you're not paralysed. It's simply that the messages from your brain to your body are very weak because of the damage."

He moves out of frame, and I hear a murmured discussion between him and James. The odd word sticks out: 'cognitive', 'function', 'future', 'hope'.

They are talking about me. Is there hope? I haven't thought about that yet. Am I going to be stuck here for ever? Am I dying? But Mister Rumble sounds so positive. He said 'repair'. My body's mending itself. They don't know how much I know, and there's no way of telling them. I want to cry. Can I cry? Well, there's a sort of moaning sound coming from somewhere, and my vision is blurring.

"It's alright." I feel a hand on mine, and I manage to clasp it.

"You're upset," says the-voice-I-love. "I'm not surprised. They're behaving as though you're not there. Mark is very, very good, but sometimes... well they all do it: they forget."

I am here, I want to say. But I know it will come out as a groan.

"I wish I could help you feel better," he says.

But he has.

I have stopped crying. I don't feel so alone now.

"You are making loads of progress. I don't think Mark expected to see your toes moving. He'll want to do some tests soon. As soon as you're ready."

He lapses into silence. I'm still holding his hand.

"Maybe I shouldn't," he murmurs to himself, and he tries to pull his hand away. I hold on for my life – my grip is stronger than he expected.

"Oh well." He sighs, and we stay like that till I hear the clip-clop of Megatron's sensible shoes.

Chapter 6

I'm running down the hall. Smoke everywhere. I must escape, but I can hear the sound of a lorry backing. It's going to crash right into the front of my house. Is it a fire engine coming to rescue me? The sound goes on and on, getting louder. My eyes are closed in expectation of the front wall of the house crashing down on me. I can hear others running up the hall behind me.

I open my eyes. There is an insistent beep coming from somewhere near me. I can hear people running. Doors being pushed open. Hard wheels on hard floors. A curtain is pulled. Low voices – indistinct. More running footsteps come close. Then silence.

There's another patient in my room. It never occurred to me that there would be someone else – I heard those voices, but they didn't make sense – I thought they were inside my head. All I have seen so far is the ceiling and people's faces when they deign to look down on me. I suppose I might be in one of those long wards I used to see in hospital dramas, but it feels like less. Probably a room with four beds in it. So there could be four people – all lying here silent. Unable to move. I find this thought unsettling, ghoulish.

Inside my head has changed, I realise. My rattled snowstorm dome has settled down, together with my see-saw emotions. The man-I-love is called James. He talks to me. Do I love him? I don't want to let go of that feeling of loving him, but I don't know how it happened. Does he love me? Another question.

The sound of people talking quietly. No words, but urgent tones. Receding footsteps.

Then the unmistakeable clip-clop of Megatron's shoes.

"We'd better move her into her own room if Doctor Park wants to do tests and therapies." I hear the disapproval in her voice.

"We don't want it disturbing the other patients. Especially not now."

There's the clatter of something at the end of my bed. More footsteps in my direction. Then a pretty face appears above me. "We're going to move you, hon. Have your own room." Her face is very white, and her eyes are dark brown. There's a hardness about her expression, as though she's become too used to people's pain.

I can hear more people around my bed. Shuffles and rattles of tubes and wires. And I'm off. My first journey in this new life. Lights give way to plain white ceiling. I see the doorway as I leave the room that I have been in for so long. The corridor is darker and I move faster. I stop and I hear the ding of a lift. Scrape of doors opening. I move into this enclosed space. Doors scrape closed. Trapped. I hate lifts. Don't know whether I'm going up or down, but that swirling feeling of body displacement is very acute in my helpless position. Ding. Doors scrape open. I'm out, and going down a lighter corridor, through a doorway, and I stop.

The white face appears above me. "Alright hon?" She moves out of sight. "We'll get you sorted out."

There's rustlings and clickings as they connect me up in my new home. The ceiling looks very similar except the lights don't seem so piercing, as though they don't want to look so deep inside me now.

It's funny. I am connected and yet I feel disconnected. It keeps happening - I want to pee, and something warm happens somewhere, and I don't want to any more. Am I stranded between life and death?

Things are quiet now, and I realise that I miss a noise that I didn't even notice before – the murmur of voices, clank of trolleys, footsteps in the distance. In here now, I become deeply aware of a hum. It must be the airconditioning, but it seems to get louder and louder. I am in a huge jet plane. Taking off. Taking off…

"…because you're special. A special case. There's so much that can be done. So much to hope for." James's voice takes on a husky note, and he stops. I can hear him breathing, and it sounds odd. Is he weeping? Is that what silent weeping sounds like?

I want to comfort him. I reach out and touch cloth.

I feel his arm jerk away. "You're awake." There's silence. He doesn't know what to say. He thought I was asleep, and doesn't know how much I heard.

"How… how are you?" His face appears looking slightly red and blotchy – maybe it's just the light and the fact he's bending over me. He manages a smile. "I'm glad you've got a new room. There's a lovely view out of the window. It's so much fresher up here."

I'd love to see the view, but the ceiling will have to do.

"They're talking of moving you into a different position so that you can see and do more. The healing has gone really well."

How do they know all this? I must have been asleep, or unconscious. I imagine being suspended from the ceiling while white-coated surgeons peer up at me, a bit like garage mechanics inspecting the underside of a car. It makes me laugh.

"Are you alright?" James's face looks down on me with a puzzled frown.

"I'm fine – just laughing," I want to say. And now I can't stop – the convulsions shake my whole body.

"I'd better get someone."

Oh James, you are so serious. Please stay. I flail about with my unseen hand and find his and hold it hard.

"Nurse," he calls. "I think you'd better check her. I think she might have had some kind of convulsion."

The sound of footsteps. A face peering down at me. She moves

31

away to read the instruments. "Mmmmh, can't see anything. I don't think it's a seizure. I'll get Doctor Park to check when he comes." She leans over me again. "Are you alright? You look OK."

I smile up at her. A baby's first achievement, and here I am doing just that.

"Well, you look happy enough."

"Sorry, I thought…"

What did you think, James?

The nurse goes away, and James sits down – out of sight, out of reach.

"I had an early start today. Six o'clock." He yawns. "There's one client." He stops himself. "Sorry, I shouldn't talk about my clients. I was forgetting. Only one person turned up to my cancer clinic today. I wonder where they all were. It will definitely get cut if no-one makes use of it." He's hurt. I can hear it in his voice.

"Anyway, Mark's coming soon, and they'll see if you're ready to be shifted into a more upright position. I'll stay with you till then. I've got nothing… on."

He stays, but he keeps his distance. What have I done? I want to hold his hand again – to feel that contact with a human being. Particularly this one.

"I cycle in at the moment. You made quite a mess of my car."

Excuse me, your car made quite a mess of me. I imagine his car on a bed with surgeons all around, probing, lifting flaps of battered plastic bumper, and I start to laugh again.

James stands up quickly and looks down on my face. I grin back up at him.

"You're laughing, so that's it, you're laughing." He smiles at last. "That was a terrible thing I just said – about the mess you made. I can't believe I said that." He starts laughing too. This is so good, this moment. Two souls in humour.

Chapter 7

Slowly, but surely, my angle tilts, and I can see sky.

"We've got your bed into a more useable position for doing the tests," I hear the gentle growl of Mister Rumble's voice. "We can see you're healing well, but we need to know how you're progressing inside."

Inside my head, you mean. But how am I to communicate if I can't speak. But just now I'm taken up with my new perspective: they have angled the top part of my bed up so that I can see out of my window. I can see the walls of the room – a plain sort-of-white colour. Clean and clinical. And now Mister Rumble comes into vision, his creased leonine face concentrating on something behind my head. He is wearing a check shirt, and I bet he's got fashionable faded jeans and moccasin type shoes on, but I'm not angled up enough to see.

There's a whirring sound and I find myself looking into a dark cavern. "Press the button when you see a little flashing light."

Button? Oh this thing in my hand. I experimentally press it, and it makes a beep. I drop it in surprise. A hand puts it back into my grasp and I hear:

"Now, when you're ready."

A flashing light appears and I press the button, but another one has already been and gone before I can press it again. I'm so slow. I'm way behind with my beeps. I've lost count of the lights that I've missed.

There is a whirr, and I can see again.

"We're going to make some sounds and I want you to press the button each time you hear one."

Somebody clicks their fingers behind my left ear. I press the button, but I'm already too late. There's another sound behind my head, and another. I keep missing them, they're too fast.

He pulls a TV screen attached to the wall so that I can just see it in the corner of my eye.

"No good," he mutters as he goes round the back of my bed.

"Can we turn her round so she's facing the screen?" This to someone I can't see. My bed turns slowly away from the window, away from the sky, until I'm facing the screen square on.

He hums to himself as he walks over to the right side of my bed, and I feel a cold flat object being slid under my hand. He lifts my hand and puts something that feels like a pencil into it, helping me to get a grip on it. But it all feels very unfamiliar – like I've never held a pencil before.

"This is a stylus and pad, and when you move the stylus it should show on the screen."

Sure enough, I can see something on the screen that looks like a wiggly line, and it moves as I move my hand. There's a clunk as I drop the stylus. He gently puts it back into my hand.

"I'm going to put up some shapes on the screen and I'll ask you to touch them with your stylus."

A square, a circle, and a triangle all appear on the screen. Large black outlines – one next to another.

I experiment with the stylus. There's a squiggle down the bottom right-hand corner of the screen.

"Right. Can you go to the circle?"

Another squiggle down on the left this time.

"Hmm, try the circle again."

I push hard and the stylus draws a jagged diagonal right across the screen, missing the circle entirely.

The screen goes blank, and then up come the shapes again. Cleaned of my attempts.

"Can you touch the triangle?"

I muster all my strength and concentration. Move carefully… and touch the square.

Exhausted, I drop the stylus and close my eyes. I just want to be left alone to look at the sky.

I hear soft footsteps, and Mister Rumble moves away from my bed to talk to someone.

"Very slow...processing...no control... responds to requests but I'm not sure how much she understands..." His hushed growl is all too audible.

"Let me try." It's the voice I want to hear. "I have an idea."

James's face appears in front of me – I want to reach out and hug him and kiss him.

"I want to try 'yes and no' with you." He looks very serious. "Can you raise your hand for yes, then don't move it for no? Let's try."

"Yes." I raise my hand just from the wrist. Hope that's enough.

"No." I do nothing.

"No." Nothing.

"Yes." Raise hand.

I see him look over at Mister Rumble, who has appeared in my vision. "Carry on," he growls.

"Does Tuesday come after Monday?" Raise hand.

"Does Friday come after Saturday?" Don't move.

James carries on with questions that become increasingly demanding, while I answer, hoping he'll stop and turn me round to look at the sky again.

"Have you read books?" Raise hand.

"Have you read Dickens?" A big favourite of mine. Raise hand.

"Is *Oliver Twist* a romantic novel?" What? No movement.

"Is *Our Mutual Friend* a romantic novel?" Why did you ask me that? I raise my hand. I suddenly feel very tired. Each time it takes a lot of effort to move my hand, and I'm realizing how many muscles are involved in that single movement.

James asks some more questions, but I simply can't respond. I close my eyes.

"I think we should stop now," says Mister Rumble from behind my bed.

They walk away.

"Cognitively, I can see that her mind is working, but her processing and motor skills… a long time…"

As I doze off I reflect that James's motor skills ran me down. If I had the energy, I'd laugh.

Chapter 8

Someone's crying.

Through the sobs I hear a disjointed monologue.

"...I can't get rid of your clothes... I can't... and here I am... what am I doing? Oh Alice if only you hadn't... and now I've done it... I've got to carry it through... don't you see? I can't leave her like this... she's got no-one... no family... nothing... I've got to... please... please..."

There's the sound of a door opening, and the monologue stops abruptly. There's the rustle of a paper tissue and the sound of a nose blowing.

Clip, clop, it's Megatron's shoes. "Are you still here Mr Penhaligon?" Her voice is full of disapproval.

"Yes I..." James croaks.

"Well I think you should go now." She pauses. "Mr Penhaligon, are you alright?"

"Yes, yes fine. Just a touch of hay fever."

At this point I pretend to wake up. I don't want James to know what I heard. God knows what he's been telling me while I've been asleep.

I make an inarticulate sound – about all I can manage at the moment.

"Hello." James is all red-eyed with his so-called hay fever. "Have a good sleep?"

I move my hand in response.

"That's great. Matron's here, I think she needs to do stuff. I'd better get off. See you tomorrow." His face disappears.

It's my turn to cry now. The one person I can communicate with is going. And I slept through all that stuff he was talking about. It's like I'm his only friend – his confessor.

Megatron moves me about like so much meat. She manages not to hurt me, but it's uncomfortable, cold, unemotional. "Bloody staffing levels," she mutters under her breath. "And now I've got this drip of a therapist hanging around. I suppose he thinks he's going to help you. Cure you. Heal you. It'll take more than a bit of talking to sort you out my girl. Running in front of his car like that. If we had fewer people like you to take care of, we'd be able to spend more time looking after the ones who really deserve it."

She plumps my leg down. Yanks the sheet over me, and leaves the room.

I miss him. I miss James. He may be obsessed with his dead Alice, but he is warm, gentle and kind. I love the feel of his hand in mine. I love his boyish face. The thought of it sends tingles down my spine. AND he's the only person who has really communicated with me for a long time. Please come back James, please come back.

Chapter 9

And he does.

Day after day he returns. And we hone our skills in communication - it's amazing what you can do with 'yes' and 'no'. I find out a lot about him. I think he forgets, sometimes, that I'm actually listening.

He talks about his clients.

I learn about the lad who always turns up late. Rebelling against overpowering parents. The lad is probably jealous of me. He knows there's someone, he's always trying to pry into James's private life.

Then there's the anxious mum of three, who comes at six thirty in the morning, and who always turns up early. I think she's in love with him – doesn't want to miss a second of her session. One time James overslept and had to answer the door in his dressing gown. She was so hurt, apparently, that it took him a lot of sessions to convince her that she was important and did have her special space in his mind.

There are more, plenty of them. But I try to forget them. I want James to myself. I want his hand, his smile, just for me.

One thing – he's never talked about Alice again. Maybe he realised that I could have been awake when he cried to her. Maybe it was just a moment, and he's got over it. Whatever, he doesn't mention her.

We sit and look out of the window, and I'm gradually being lifted into an upright position. My head is healing, and I'm beginning to be able to move it from side to side.

I can look at him now, when I choose, and I can use my facial expressions and semi-comprehensible grunts to communicate at a deeper level.

Then comes the day when I can see far enough out of the window to see the ground – far below me in my fifth-storey room.

It comes as a shock that just past the car park is a graveyard. James is sitting by my bed and I reach out and give his hand a squeeze. We sit looking out at it together in silence for a long time. Then James sighs, lets go of my hand and gets up and walks to the window. I wonder if she's buried there. As I look at his back I can feel his loneliness.

Chapter 10

Far from just wriggling my toes, I can move my legs now. They are stiff and reluctant, and every time I start in the morning it feels like I've never done it before. But each time I get them moving just that bit quicker.

My arms are moving freely, if a bit feebly, but my grip is very uncontrolled, and eating is a long messy work in progress.

I long to get out of bed, but my core strength is too weak at the moment. I'd just flop over like a rag doll. And there's the ataxia – that horrible uncertainty that my muscles might suddenly fail completely without any warning.

Most of my tubes have come out – just the odd thing gets attached from time to time, but now I can feed myself...

Learning to swallow again was scary and uncomfortable. I kept feeling I was going to choke. Something I always took for granted became a horrible convulsive experience for a time.

"Sausage, beans and mash." James has a smile on his face as he helps me get the spoon to my mouth.

"I had almost the same at home yesterday."

I wonder if he feeds himself properly. He is so thin.

"A bit of mustard really helps with the sausages." He bends down and picks up a pot of Colman's. "Would you like?"

I manage a nod. The hospital food tends to be a bit bland. No exotic flavours here, but mustard! As I fork in a lump of sausage primed with mustard, I wonder how he knew. Does he always walk around with a pot of mustard in his pocket, on the off-chance that there'll be a sausage? The heat and strength of flavour make me choke a little, and James looks concerned, but I get it down and there's a warm feeling inside that comes from the mustard. Or does it?

"Ow deed ooh oh?" I ask, hoping he might pick my meaning.

"I checked the menu yesterday, but it's always sausages on a

Thursday."

Work out the week by the food, I think. Also I'm working out the rhythm of James's visiting times, which fluctuate each day according to what he's doing, both in and out of the hospital.

This morning they washed my hair, which has grown quite a bit since I came into hospital. I know it is nice hair – dare I say beautiful? James reaches out and touches it. Then strokes it, and I feel an awakening down in my body. I want to hold him, and him to hold me. He strokes the side of my face with the back of his hand, and I reach out and hold it there.

"I miss you when I'm at home." So close, so warm. "I'd like to see you more, but…" He shrugs his shoulders, letting go of my hand. He gets up and walks to the window. That forlorn, thin back. If only I could get out of bed and go to him. Hug him.

He turns, his face smiling. "Next week we're going to try and get you out of bed." He walks over to me. "I've got to go now. See you tomorrow."

I want to cry. I want to stop him from coming in and out of my life. The gaps between seeing him are long and painful. Bed sores, constipation, injections, and the awful Megatron.

"Goodbye."

Chapter 11

I wake up. Something's wrong, very wrong. I can hear creaks and groans coming from above me, and a smell of burning rubber. I can hear Mum stirring in the next room. I'm too scared to speak, too scared to cry out.

Mum sounds worried, "What's that smell Alf? What's going on? I can smell burning rubber."

There's a scrambling noise, and then I hear Dad grunting, "It's the middle-of-the-fucking-night."

"There's something wrong Alf." I hear Mum's urgent voice. "Get up, get up! Oh I'm going out to have a look." I hear the door click open, and footsteps in the hall, then coughing. Mum's voice is much louder now. "There's smoke everywhere. Quick get up, check the children. I think there's a fire."

There's a groaning noise, then a thump as Dad falls out of bed. "What the...?"

More scrambling, my door opens. "Mel, get up quick!" Her voice is urgent, I'm out of bed and on my feet, reaching for my dressing gown.

"Where are Peter, Max and Chris?" I hear Dad calling from down the hall.

"God, they're up the top with their cousins!" My mum is sounding panicky now. "We should wake everybody up! Why can't we hear anyone else? You go and look, Alf, and I'll call the fire..."

There is a huge crash, and the ceiling gives way just along the hall. I can hear the roaring now, and can feel the heat coming at me from the furnace that was my home. Another crash, and the ceiling, just to our left, gives way, sending sparks into our frightened faces. We pause, frozen in panic. We can hear screams now, over the noise of the disintegrating house. The rest of our family is trapped at the top of the house. More smoke billows

43

out of the inferno, masking everything around us, and making us choke and stagger.

"Quick!" Mum takes me by the hand, dragging me in the direction of the front door. Dad stands helpless looking in the direction of what had once been the stairs.

"Alf! Alf!" Mum screams. "We've got to get out!" The ceiling comes down between us, leaving Dad stranded behind burning wreckage.

Crying with anguish, she pulls me towards the front door. Coughing and choking, feeling like our skin is burning off the backs of our legs, we scramble and stagger to the door. Locked! The key is back in Mum and Dad's bedroom. A Chubb lock is going to kill us.

"Quick, the loo!" Mum turns right and into the downstairs cloakroom, the fire hasn't reached that yet. The window is high but big enough for us to clamber through. Stuck! The window won't open, she grabs a shoe from the rack and pounds at the glass, smashing it, the fragments spraying down on us. Urgently mum pushes me up to the window, I struggle through, jagged pieces of glass cutting my hands. I land outside awkwardly and sit on the gravel clutching my ankle with bleeding hands. Mum comes through in a shower of glass, blood streaming from her hands and knees.

I look up, the whole house is ablaze – a terrifying inferno. I can hear the sirens now.

"Get away from the house. Get back." Mum's voice is desperate above the roaring, crackling and crashing. I can hear the house collapsing inside. Where are my brothers, my cousins, my aunts and uncles? And Dad? Smoke is beginning to pour from the toilet window, surely he'll come out. As I back away, staring at the window, there is another crash, and the front door falls out. Smoke and flames pour out into the darkness, and there, stumbling through the gap is my dad, his clothes ablaze.

Choking, his arms flailing, he staggers down the drive towards the flashing lights of a fire engine that has just screeched to a halt on the front drive. Firemen jump out with blankets, and for a moment he disappears, smothered by the rescuers, then I hear him screaming, "My boys, my family they're all stuck up the top!"

I look up at the top floor of the house, hoping to see some sign of life, but it is all flames. Every window a furnace. Then with a shuddering crash the roof gives way, collapsing into the house. There is no chance now of any escape. The firemen are rapidly pulling out their hoses, getting the ladders up as close as they dare. There are three engines now, and another one round the back. Is there hope there? Has anyone got out of the back of the house? A firemen returns, his face saying it all. One big family – now just a few singed remnants being bundled into an ambulance. Stunned, dead inside. Unbelieving. Silent.

Chapter 12

Sunshine, blessed sunshine on my face. After what seems like months of incarceration, I am out. A warm breeze coming up the coast is caressing my skin, bringing it back to life. The rehab hospital garden is like a marvellous oasis to me. Every plant, flower, tree a revelation to my neon-tired eyes. I drink it in, gratefully. Birds fly down and land near me. A blackbird's feathers glint in the sun, giving them colours that I'd never noticed before. I can hear the seagulls above the traffic calling in that forever-yearning way. The sea, how I long for it. To put my toes in the water. Stand and feel the rhythmic tug of the waves round my ankles.

I look down at my knees and find myself back with harsh reality. I can't walk. I can't talk. I am just learning to use my fingers clumsily – my fine motor skills coming back in dribs and drabs. My obtuse and reluctant body resisting every attempt I make to control it. The agony of frustration that overwhelms me sometimes, making me cry like a baby. Helpless.

Still, here I am. Sitting up in a wheelchair, my hand on an iPad, able to communicate at last, if slowly. I feel like I'm daft as my mind races ahead of my disobedient fingers, but as I remember the dream I had last night, I realise that I've cheated death for a second time, and that feeling of something round the corner stays with me – optimism. I know I'm lucky – so many people would give their eye teeth, their balance and their speech, to have that hope that lives in my heart.

Andy's voice interrupts my reverie. "James will be here in a minute, and we can start your new exercises. You have made so much progress." Andy is my physio at the rehabilitation centre. I wonder if he is joking about my progress – I feel like I'm getting nowhere. "Soon you can leave here, once we have got you to stand." Why does he always have to go on about standing? The very thought of it makes me feel sick and dizzy. The ground is such a long way away that I don't dare to look down out of my wheelchair. An abyss is waiting under the wheels.

There is something else too, that's been on my mind and has resurfaced now to haunt me: where will I live when I leave hospital? It all feels so cold and cruel now, after my moment of sunshine in the hospital garden.

"Hello." I hear James's voice behind me and I turn carefully to look into his eyes - holding his gaze for a moment. He looks tired, distracted. I notice creases in his face that I haven't seen before.

Have I done this to him? I have been so much work for him.

I slowly type 'love you' into my iPad and show it to him, trying to screen it from Andy's gaze.

"Can we have a moment alone?" he says to Andy.

Andy backs off looking slightly surprised. "A few minutes, and then we must get started. I'll just go and check…"

James squats down and takes my hands. He looks into my eyes and says quietly, "I've been thinking, this is all very difficult, but… it's all… I'm finding it hard coming here to see you and help you. I go home and feel so… lonely. I can't sleep. And there's my cl… people to see, and…"

I look down at our hands. "Dend yee mee." (*Then leave me.*) I feel the tears start to come.

He shakes my hands, trying get me to look at him. "No, no it's not like that. I don't want to leave you. I want… you to come and stay at my place so I can look after you. I've lain awake at night thinking about this. I don't know how we can manage, but I want to try."

I look him full in the face, smiling, tearful, and nod. I take my left hand away from his and type. "Yes."

He gives a big sigh and his tired face brightens for a moment. "You're so… I…" He looks over his shoulder, and nods to Andy who is standing in the doorway. "Right, Andy's waiting, we'd better get started."

They wheel me to one of the physio rooms, and prepare to get me out of the sanctuary of my wheelchair.

"OK let's do this very slowly and carefully," says Andy. "You take one elbow, James, and I'll take the other."

The ground opens up in front of me – an impossible chasm. Gales blow at my head, my stomach disappears and there is nothing between my heavy teeming brain and my weak spindly legs.

"Tant doo eet," I whimper. (*Can't do it*)

"We've got you, you can't fall."

The world plunges and wavers, the chasm remains, but somehow a distant memory tells me I can move my leg. Right leg first – lift. Nothing. Big effort – tiny shuffle forward.

"Well done, well done. Now the right leg."

But I've just done the right leg. Panic takes over. My brain is back to front – wrong way round. I feel sick, and suddenly weak all over. I am falling, falling.

"Eel it". (*Feel sick*)

"What did she say?"

"I think she's going to be sick."

They let me down into my wheelchair, but the room still swims in front of my eyes – the floor is miles away, and everything has an odd echo as though I am in some vast cave. My stomach returns but with it is the feeling of being impossibly full. Nausea comes quickly – I try to hold on, but the contents of my overburdened stomach spill out into the bowl in front of me. I feel a cool flannel on my forehead, as someone mops my face. I gradually begin to calm down in the security of my chair, and I look up to see James's kind troubled face.

Andy kneels down in front of me. "We've got to keep trying," he says. "You took a step. I know it made you sick but your brain

49

has got to work this out – build new pathways. I know it seems impossible, but I have seen this before, and you can get through it. I know it's a mountain to climb." He comes out with all this as if it is an ill-prepared speech to a class of six-year-olds. "See you tomorrow."

I shudder – they can't possibly expect me to do this again. Can they?

Next day, the day after, and on and on we try. Always encouraging, but I am getting nowhere. It is always the same: the chasm opens up and I feel like I'm falling, falling. The dizziness, the nausea, and now the frustration.

Then one day I decide to take my life in my own hands. I will do it, I will take that step. Mark and James are on either side of me, ready to support, when unexpectedly I lurch forward, catching them unawares. I fail to catch hold of the walking frame and the floor comes up to meet me with surprising speed. My head hits something hard. Everything goes black and in the distance I can hear the roar of voices, as though going away down a long corridor. Then, nothing. Silence.

The Dreamhouse

I

The house is strangely familiar. I'm standing in a long hall with doors on both sides leading to various rooms – rooms that I'm sure I've been in before. And at the end of the hall is a broad imposing staircase with dark wooden banisters – Victorian I suppose. I suspect that if I go up that staircase I will find an infinite number of halls and doors leading to an infinite number of rooms, and it will take me forever to see them all – in fact, I never will. I'm not ready for that staircase and all that infinity, so I go to the first door on the right, open it, and walk into the room.

I wish I hadn't.

It is a large circular chamber and placed round the walls are dark objects whose shapes are difficult to make out in the gloomy light. In the middle is a spiral staircase which goes up and up and disappears into the darkness above. It descends as well, going down into the depths below. I find myself drawn to the objects at the edge of the room. They give off a heavy sense of something I don't want to see, and yet, and yet I'm terribly attracted to them.

They are things that have never been forgiven. I don't want to know them any more, but at the same time I'm addicted to them. The pain of that hurt, that slight, that insult, never forgotten, never forgiven. Held on to for ever. That glorious pain, like holding the wrong end of a burning hot poker. 'Hold it, hold it tight Melissa. Feel it burn into your flesh.' I love the pain of holding on to unforgiveness. All those precious wounds. I can see them and feel them all at once in this room. I don't ever want to let go of them – can't let go of them.

'He said this, she said that, they must hate me – how can they?'

And childhood: 'They made me do this, they never listened, they didn't look after me, they didn't care.'

I wander round this room, horribly enthralled, wanting, yearning to touch each wound as though it's a blessing.

Ah, there's a really powerful one: 'Nobody understands me!'

And now I want to rend these hurts - to tear them apart. But it's me that I would hurt. I never get too close as I wander round the room. The objects are shrouded in a mist, which makes them seem attractive from a distance, but I don't want to see them too clearly. I daren't. I would be lost forever in the fascination of my hurts, never to see another room. Never to move on.

II

I'm out of the door before I know it, and I have closed it with a sudden desire to get on and explore this vast house.

I open the next door on the right and nearly stumble into a huge dark hole, just catching hold of the door frame in time. This room is circular too, and so large that it is hard to see the other side in the sepulchral gloom. There is a bit of floor going right round the circumference of this huge chamber - just enough to get round if I keep my back pressed against the wall. My fear of heights nearly makes me leave the room and carry on with my exploration. Why risk my neck in this seemingly empty and dangerous space when there is so much more to see?

I blink, and in that moment the room is transformed. There is a beautiful oak floor running from the lip on which I'm standing, and reaching right over to the other side. A blue glow lights the room up making it feel fresh, creative, and I can hear the sound of the sea. I am very attracted by this room now, wanting nothing more than to go right to the centre into that blue light, and feel the fresh seaside air on my face. I pause, taking all this in and wondering how it could be safe. Then I take a step onto the oak, ready to jump back if it gives way.

The floor is firm and smooth under my bare feet. I can feel the pulse of old, old wood - warm with its still-retained life. I can see something in the middle of the room, and as I get closer, walking slowly and carefully, I see that it is a small table with a polished top and slim turned legs. The wood has a reddish hue, like cherry, giving it an inviting warmth, and there is a wooden chair by it which looks old and comfortable. I feel invited to sit in this chair, and as I move to do so a sheet of paper appears on the surface of the table, with a pen made of some rare wood. I sit down and start to write. I write whatever comes into my head, and as I look down at the paper in front of me, I realise I am writing a great story. Something I never imagined I would do. Never.

Time passes and I just bask in this lovely room with its peaceful sounds of the sea and its gentle blue light. I have finished the story, and look at it with amazement – where did that come from? Then over my shoulder I feel a presence, a person who knows me. Can I trust them with this new story of mine?

The words I hear are harsh and destructive – no encouragement, and I feel a terrible sinking sensation in my stomach. Simultaneously the table begins to disintegrate. My story falls to the floor now beyond my reach and to my horror the floor itself starts to collapse. The trusty old oak floorboards rot in front of my eyes and I leap up just as my chair gives way and stagger back, keeping away from the widening circle of darkness in front of me. I must get back to the door and I turn and flee as the rotting boards give way behind me, just making it to the wall in time as the entire floor disappears into the chasm leaving just the lip round the edge of the room. I cling to the wall, I can't see the door and I turn round in the darkness – just me, this lip, and the wall.

I've got to find a way out of here, but the door has disappeared. In the darkness and confusion I must have gone to the wrong side of the room. I can't stand this aloneness on a ledge with a huge fall below me. I wobble, my knees start to give way, I cling to the wall but I'm facing away from it so there is no proper grip. Everything starts to rock, the wall becomes slimy – no grip at all, and I slide away from it and into the void.

III

I am falling. Am I Alice? But this is no rabbit hole, no certainty that something weird and comforting will happen. I pass something sticking out and grab hold of it. In the gloom I can see it's a knife with writing on it.

'Cut yourself, then you will feel better', it says.

I'm tempted but fortunately my hands are still so slippery from the slimy wall that I drop it and it disappears into the gloom below without a sound. I feel sick – I'm sure I'm going to be sick before I hit the bottom of this pit, and die in a heap of crushed bones and ruptured flesh. I try to scream, but no sound comes out – I'm stuck in this nightmare.

Down, down I fall. It gradually gets lighter and lighter, and then, I see the glint of something coming up fast to meet me.

I hit the water hard – it stings my feet, and feels very cold as I go down deep. I can't breathe. I struggle up through the weight of the water. I can see light above me – blue. Keep going up and up – I will breathe in water at any moment and then I will drown. The light seems overpowering as I reach the surface, gasping and flailing. Exhausted, exuberant – I'm alive!

I'm in a pool with green banks all around, and trees in what looks like a garden. I struggle to the bank and haul myself out to flop on the grassy slope and feel the sun on my skin, warming and drying me. As I stretch my arms out to feel the soft grass and the warmth of the sun, my hand comes into contact with something sharp. I feel it prick my skin and I recoil, bringing my hand in front of my eyes to look at the damage. There is a small cut on the back of my hand and blood is coming out of it in tiny droplets. I suck the wound and taste my own blood. Slightly salty. The bleeding stops and I raise myself on my elbow to see what had cut me. There lying on the grass is the knife.

'*Cut yourself*'.

Once again I feel tempted, but overcoming my urge for self harm I take the knife by the handle and fling it into the pool where it disappears with a plop going down to unknown depths.

Safe at last. Safe from myself, I snuggle down into the luxurious warm grass and look up into the sky. The clear blueness of it and the gentle warmth coming down from it remind me of mornings spent on the beach by the Mediterranean sea, when all I had to think about was where the next meal was coming from. After a while, I realise that I'm hungry. It's a curious kind of hunger – more a restless need to find something to feed me. I get up from my cosy grass-bed and look around. I am in the Night Garden, I am in C.S. Lewis's Garden Between Worlds, I am in the Garden of Eden. Dark and light, mysterious and welcoming, it draws me on into its heart.

As I walk, I realise that it is all very familiar. It is like the garden of my childhood – dreamt or remembered. Wide sweeping lawns and cedar trees giving aromatic shade. High borders of rhododendrons with their bright colours, and old pink roses with such sweet scent. Every now and then I catch a glimpse of some great tree – a Scots pine looking top heavy, a glorious copper beech, and a very climbable yew tree. As I wander down the lawns guided on my way by impregnable borders I come upon an apple orchard. Most of the trees are quite small, but all are old. In the centre is a much larger tree with big red and green apples. I want one of these apples but because of the height of the branches I have to reach up to grab hold of one. It comes away from the branch with a sudden movement, sending dry bits of leaf and dead wood floating down on me. I brush the detritus from my face and hair and take a bite. The apple is juicy, refreshing and slightly bitter. When I was young I was told to let the fruit ripen, but I always liked the bitterness of fruit before its time. Is this the tree of life? I ponder. Is this the fruit I wasn't supposed to eat? But if so, where's the serpent?

At that moment I am startled by a sudden rush of colour as a large bird glides past me and up into the high trees surrounding the orchard. I follow the direction of its flight, longing to see it more clearly. But it is gone – swallowed up in the verdant forest that I now see is on every side of the garden.

I walk on, munching the apple, and feeling small but protected in this mother of gardens. So it comes as a shock when I round a corner and come across an impenetrable barrier of fallen trees. Six great elms lie prone on the ground in a row, their roots pointing up to the sky, the fresh earth still dangling from their fibrous ends. The trees lie long and straight, the bark ridged and peppery brown. I am tempted to clamber up onto the trunk of the nearest tree and go back to my childhood, playing games – imagining I'm in a space rocket going to Mars. I resist. I'm an adult now, even if I feel small. I can't play these games any more, and anyway, I'm sad to see these wonderful trees brought so low to die and rot on the ground.

As I gaze at them wondering what brought them down, and how I am going to get round them, I become aware of a presence behind me. I turn to see a boy of about fifteen. He is looking straight at me with his hands behind his back. His face is covered by a white mask with an 'O' shape for a mouth. But looking through the mask his eyes are cold as they survey me. He makes me feel as if I have no clothes on, and I just want to run and hide from him, but I am rooted to the spot – mesmerized. Slowly, he brings his right hand round from behind his back. It is holding a knife – that knife, and I wonder how he managed to get it from the bottom of the pool. I reach forward and take the knife from him. I notice that he has been holding the blade and that blood drips from his hand onto the grass, staining it red. I look at the blade and 'Cut yourself' is still visible through the blood, then I turn it over to see more writing: 'This knife cuts both ways'. I look up again but the youth has disappeared leaving a small pool of red on the green grass, and an impression of his eyes - still staring. The knife tempts me. I hold out my arm. *'Then you will feel better.'* But I'm in a place before all that. I'm back in a safe world before the happening, before I lost my nerve to live, before all my anger and my rage. My take on the world.

I turn and plunge the knife into the trunk of the great elm next to me. My fury drives it deep, and in that moment I hear the grinding of worlds warping - like the sound of huge trees splitting. The garden changes shape before my eyes - colours pressed together like flowing paint. Clear at first and then becoming blurred as they come too close to see. I am swallowed up. The massive grating, squealing sound overpowers all else and I give myself up to be ground between dimensions - pummelled into another existence.

All colours make white - all colours make black!

IV

It's dark, and all I can see is a small pool of light coming up from the floor. As my eyes begin to focus, I find that I am at the top of a spiral staircase and that it leads down through mist towards the light. I am still holding the knife, and it dawns on me that I can't just get rid of it. That until I have mastered it, it will always come back to me, and I will never return to that room where I can write my story. I so want to be there again, with the blue light and the writing table. But it is a dangerous place for me now - at any moment that floor could give way.

These stairs seem solid enough though, so I go down them and into the gloom. At least I've got the knife!

I grasp the rail of the spiral staircase and begin my descent. There is an eerie feeling of being suspended high above nothingness. Through the mist that surrounds me I can see no end to this climb down. The stairs recede below me, turning silver in the cloudy light. There is no visible support for this staircase, just the steps and the rail spiralling down. I grip the rail tightly, scared of falling over the side into nothingness. After a while my feet start to get sore from the metal steps, my arm aches from the tension of gripping the rail, and I begin to wonder when this will end. Then I hear faint sounds below me. At first they sounds like a wind, low and echoing round this cavernous void. But as I get closer I can hear many voices:- calling, pleading, moaning, laughing, - and I realise that I am ending up back in the room of unforgiveness, and it is a place of madness. These demanding voices cajoling, mocking, accusing. Seen from the outside like this, they now seem very unattractive. Why was I ever taken in by them?

At last I am nearing the floor, which I now can see is stained with tears. Dark streaks and salty deposits all over what was once a beautiful elm floor. And as I walk towards the wall of this circular room, the shapes making these mad sounds come into focus for the first time.

They are dark green plants with huge black flowers, their stems covered in spikes and bristles. The black petals are hard and shiny, so unlike the soft velvety surface of a natural flower. I get close enough to touch one of these plants and I see how repulsive it is, gleaming in the half-light. It is saying how left out it feels, never included, never accepted, always alone. "Nobody loves me, nobody cares..." I want to hear no more and I plunge the knife right into the centre of the black flower. There is a shriek, followed by rustling and creaking and the flower starts growing. Before I stabbed it, it came up to my shoulder; now I see it growing up the wall to tower above me, leaning over me, threatening me.

I stagger back and look down at my left arm which is starting to sting. To my horror it is bleeding. I must have cut myself when I stabbed the flower. *This knife cuts both ways.* The other plants all start to lean towards me, mocking me. "Stab us, cut us," they say, "and see what happens." One revolting creeper sends out a tendril to brush my face. It is prickly and slimy and I lash out at it with the knife. The end of the tendril falls to the floor and starts to grow right by my feet. I feel my left arm sting again and look down to see another cut just below the first one. If I carry on like this I will end up cutting my wrist. I must get out. There is no way I can sort out this unforgiven room. I look round the walls for the door, but all I can see are these shiny black flowers lining the walls. The only way out is in the centre of the room, so I turn and make for the spiral staircase, feeling the brush of hairy tendrils on my back.

I reach the stairs and start to climb, but then it dawns on me that if I go back up I will never get out. I will be stuck with this knife and this horrible resentment for ever. Just going round in circles.

No. I must go down below the room, and into the dark. However frightening it is, it's the only way out. The metal spiral staircase changes into a stone one with no handrail as I descend below floor level. It is wet under my feet, and I can't see anything at all in the gloom below. I half stagger, half slip down the cold stone steps, wondering if I'm just going to fall off the edge and into oblivion. My head is below the floor of the room of unforgiveness now, and all is dark down here. The only light is from the room above, and it is faint so I can't see far into the gloom. I wonder how much farther I am going to have to creep down into this dark damp cave, when my feet find no more steps, but just what feels like damp earth. I step cautiously away from the stone stairs and I am blind. I stop to try and get my bearings. There is a smell of damp earth down here, and a faint rustle and creak of something moving in the gentle cool breeze that I can now feel on my face. Amidst all the fear of the unknown that surrounds me I feel my heart leap – there must be a way out down here. That breeze must come from somewhere. Maybe I can get back into that beautiful garden. But I'm still holding the knife, and I don't want to let go of it. I can't let go of it.

With my left arm stretched out in front of me I walk slowly forward in the direction I feel this breeze is coming from. All my senses are heightened by this blindness. I can feel every little lump of mud beneath my feet, hear every noise – and there is noise. What had sounded like a rustle is clearly more like the sound of many damp things rubbing against each other. My mind conjures up horrible images of the limbs of dead people, hanging from the ceiling of this dark cavern, all gently swaying in the wind. So it is almost a relief when I feel something fibrous with my hand. A root. It must be a root! I walk slowly forward and feel another, then another. But after a few steps they are getting thicker and longer and are really starting to block my way. If I'm going to get out of here I'm going to have to hack my way out. I feel the knife in my hand. Will it just cut me as I cut the roots? I'm going to have to try, so I cautiously take hold of the nearest root and take the knife and start to hack at it. It's much tougher than I expected. The knife feels blunt, and I have to make a sawing motion to feel like I'm having any affect. Just when I think that I'm getting nowhere I feel the root come away in my hand and simultaneously I hear a thump and a shriek from the room above.

The surprise makes me drop the knife, and as I grope down in the dark, it dawns on me that these are the roots of the ghastly black flowers in the room of unforgiveness. There's a stinging feeling on my left arm – I must have cut myself. I feel it to see if I'm bleeding and my arm is wet, but I can't be sure whether it's the moisture of this damp place that covers me, or whether it's my blood.

I can't find the knife. I'm blind in this darkness and I'm starting to panic.

"Don't move from this spot," I say to myself. "You'll never find it if you move." So I keep my feet as much in the same place as possible and crouch down, swinging my right arm around in a wide arc. It can't have gone far. My hand brushes against something slimy that moves, and I jerk back, almost falling over. I want to scream but no sound comes out of my mouth. Stuck here in the dark. Alone. I sit down and something sharp against my thigh makes me get up again. I put my hand on it – it's the knife.

I must stand up, face the breeze, and cut my way out of here. I might find my left arm hacked to pieces but it's the only way. Slowly I move forward, cutting through one root and then another in a seemingly endless process. The satisfaction of hearing the plants above me shriek and fall keeps me going, along with the knowledge that it can't be far to the edge of the room. And then I'll get out. It's merciless, hard work, and each time I cut through another root I wonder if my left arm has another gash in it. I haven't felt anything since it stung the first time, and I am beginning to wonder whether I imagined it. I'm making progress here, the breeze is getting stronger, and I can hear something else mixed in with the rubbery creaking of the roots. It's a rhythmic lulling sound that calls up faint memories. In this dark hell I find it hard to recall anything good in my mind, so fixed am I on survival and escape. The earth is feeling different beneath my feet – softer, dryer, sandier. And then it comes to me. I'm hearing the sea.

But there are still some particularly tough roots to cut through, and my arm's getting very tired. I hack and hack, and two more go, and then it feels as if I have only one root to go, but this one is really stubborn, and the knife feels blunter than ever, in fact it feels like it's changing shape. There are still some strands of this root to cut through, but what I'm holding doesn't feel like a knife at all. In desperation I wrench and pull at the root, but it won't break. I feel the knife, careful not to cut myself: most of its length is like a smooth stem, but at one end there's a ring and the other end sticks out proud of the stem and is serrated. I put this against the first strand of root and saw. It comes away. I do the

62

same again, and again until I hear a loud shriek and a thump as the plant in the room above me falls to the floor, and I stumble out into water.

V

It laps round my ankles, cool. I can smell the salt, but still I can see nothing. I look up – it's pitch black. Has all sight gone from my world? Am I to be blind for ever? I feel the tears in my eyes, and I just want to give up. But something inside me says otherwise:

"Sing in the dark," it says. So I start to sing. It's a strange improvised song without words, a sort of lament. A grieving lullaby for the child I never had. It's almost as if someone else were singing it. My love, my child.

As I sing and look up a tiny light appears above me, then another and another. Stars are lighting up my sky, and I remember a childhood book: big bear carries out little bear, 'I give you the moon'.

And so I sing for the moon in a voice that is deep, rich, and resonant, and out comes a huge harvest moon, low on the horizon. An orange moon that turns to gold and then to silver as it climbs up into the sky. And from this shining moon I can see the rippling of the waves, a gentle sea. It's warm and I'm standing on the edge of it, revelling in its peacefulness. I look behind me and the root-filled horror has gone. In its stead is a long sandy beach surrounded by pine trees. To my right and left the sand curls forward into the sea, making a protective bay, and I am held in its arms.

My arm! I look down at my left arm, fearing what I might see, but there are no cuts on it, just some abrasions that look like they might be caused by a very blunt saw. It feels bruised but otherwise undamaged. I look at my right hand and instead of holding a knife, I'm grasping a large bronze key, about nine inches long.

The sort that would open the door of some ancient castle. The serrations at the lock end must be what caused the scratches on my arm, but they are also what finally hacked through the last root and released me. Is this paradise? This place that I have escaped to? Or is it the edge of my mind? Should I plunge forward and dare to dive down into my depths? Or should I go back up the beach, through the trees and find a lock for this key? The sea invites me with its warm lulling rhythm, but I look at the key and wonder.

Turning round, I scan the beach for an entrance into the wood, and just to the left I can make out a break in the trees. Reluctantly, I walk up the beach away from the inviting waters, and feeling the sand between my toes, I make my way towards the gap. There is a path through the pine wood. The roots stand proud of the sand in places, giving a feeling of children's-book fantasy. In the moonlight the sand looks like snow, and the trees curl in on either side of the path. As I look up at them I feel very small, like I'm a child. Quietly, feeling as though I'm trespassing, I creep up the path trying not make a sound. A fawn appears just ahead of me, looks surprised for a moment and then trots off into the trees. I become aware of a shadow above me, and an owl silently glides up the path in front of me – a mysterious magical creature. The mossy lumps in the banks on either side of me make curious sculptures, their shadows made sharp by the cold light of the moon. And the smell, that resonant aroma of pine, is intoxicating.

I know in my heart that I will come back this way to the beach, but first I must open a door with this heavy bronze key. I hold it tightly, as if my life depended on it.

The path takes me deeper into the wood and it's almost impossible now to imagine that I could be so close to the sea. Slightly uphill all the time, it twists and turns, and the sand is laced with pine needles making the walking slightly prickly. It feels like it will go on for ever, so it's a shock when I come into a large sandy clearing and there before me is a house. Stone built, with flying buttresses and towers, arched windows and decorative doorways, it could be a grand mansion except it is too small. Like all these ideas were packed into a child's space – a folly.

I walk down the sandy slope towards the front door, and there, sitting in an armchair beside it, is an old woman. As I get closer, I half recognise her but cannot think from where. She is dressed in dark flowing clothes, and has large ornate rings on her crooked fingers. She looks straight at me with piercing eyes, her face is neither smiling nor frowning, and her mouth hangs open slightly in the shape of an 'O'. I cannot decide whether she is a witch or a wise woman. I can feel her power, and it makes me frightened. I fear that whatever she says will affect me, and it will be hard to resist her and go my own way. Can I trust her? Well, this is the only way into the house so I will have to go past her.

I hold out my hand with the key in it: "I have a key." My voice sounds tremulous and childish.

"Yes," she says.

"I... I think this is right..."

There is a small low table in front of her with an old-fashioned alarm clock on it. She looks at it, frowns and says, "Well, it is time to... go." Her voice sounds sad, as though she has no wish to hurt me, and she gets up stiffly from her armchair, goes to the front door and opens it.

I murmur "Thanks" as I pass her, go through the doorway and beyond the reach of her power.

VI

I am back in the same hallway that I started in. The serried ranks of doors on both sides with the massive staircase at the end leading to infinity. There is a difference though. Everything is much bigger. The doors are more than twice my height, and if I

65

reach up I will just be able turn the handles. That is why the key is so big, I realise. Then I look down at my hands and I see the hands of a child. Of course, I have become a child. Will I enter the Kingdom of Heaven? Well, I know I want to go back to that beach, and that felt like paradise. So maybe?

I know I don't want to go through the first door on my right. No, I'm not making that mistake again. So I look to the left, and as I look at the high door I read the words 'Growth Room One' in faded black printed across the old worn wood. I turn the handle, it is hard for my little hand but I grip tight and feel it click. The door doesn't budge. It's locked. So this must be the time to use my key. Using both hands I heft the key up and into the keyhole below the handle. The key won't turn. I pull it out a bit to see if that makes any difference. No good. I push it in harder, the key works this time, and the lock clicks open. I turn the handle and go in.

It is quite a small room – even though I am child-size it feels disappointingly small. It is completely empty. Just blank walls and ceiling. There is no window. The light comes from the walls which are painted a gentle white. The floor, which is wooden, is also painted white. The door closes behind me and I suddenly feel trapped. Claustrophobia has always been a problem for me. I begin to panic, but somewhere inside there's a voice saying 'Calm down, breathe. Listen.'

To start with all I can hear is my rapid heartbeat pounding in my head, but as I calm down I can hear a faint roar – a river inside me? Quieter still there is a high-pitched whine – the sound of my nervous system working ceaselessly. I wonder what else I will uncover, what other secret sounds I've been carrying around with me. Then I hear it: faint laughter. Is it coming from inside, or from the walls? Gradually the sound grows and I can hear talking. It sounds warm and genial – grown-ups having a gentle time together. The voices sound familiar, taking me back to...

about the age I seem to be now. It sounds like my family, all aunts and uncles, cousins, parents, brothers, gathered together for some occasion. Christmas? I long to be with them, to see their faces again. I go to press my ear against the wall, and to my amazement the wall feels like it's made of some silky material and I just find myself pushing through it as if it were soft silky jelly.

I'm in the sitting room with them. Our comfy old sitting room just as it was when I was little. The other children are gathered round the fireplace, sitting on the floor and playing Monopoly. The grown-ups are seated in the old tatty armchairs, and on the sofa with the arm that won't stay up any more. Talking, laughing, getting on in a way that only families do when they are at ease with themselves. The curtains are drawn across the French windows that I know will lead to the steps up to the croquet lawn. I look round for the wall I've just come through and there is the ornate framed print of *The Battle of San Romano* by Uccello. I am home.

"There you are Mel, come on, come and join us. Have you been hiding behind the curtains again, playing with your dollies?" My auntie Doris has turned round and seen me. She beckons me over and I half stumble into the circle of parents and children, and plump myself down on my daddy's knee. He gives me a squeeze, and an affectionate kiss on my head and the other adults turn round to look at me. Love fills their faces, but I can see there is some concern there too. "Always playing on your own, such an imagination. Where will you end up?" My dad hands me over to Mum who gives me another hug, and I can feel tears in my eyes. I am loved. I know it then – gratitude. I am lucky. I may have lost most of my family all those years ago, it may have become dysfunctional and disconnected, but I was loved. I had this family, and I will always have it inside me. Thank you, thank you, thank you!

I weep then, letting all my emotion pour out, and as I do so the picture fades and I find myself back in the white room. Back with myself. But I'm feeling a bit different - warmer inside. The tears may have regret in them, but there's a large portion of gratitude, and a feeling of having been so lucky.

I long to be back there. It was such a fleeting visit, just a taste of things past. The room is silent again, just the sounds of my alive body. But there is a smell, faint to start with, but getting stronger. Pencil shavings. It brings back memories of school. I shiver. School, that ghastly place, that prison where I was forced to waste so much of my early life. And I can hear something new now, the faint sound of crying. It pulls me, tugs at my heart, and it's coming from the wall straight ahead. I have to go and comfort that poor soul, so I walk to the wall expecting to go straight through, but I nearly bash my nose on its solid surface. My hands sting where I slap them on the plaster. The crying goes on. Louder now. Sobbing, lonely crying. I can't bear it. I have to get to the poor soul who is so sad, so alone. I look round the room, but the only way out is the door in the opposite wall. If I go out, will I lose track of the crying? I couldn't bear that - I must go and comfort whoever it is. I go to the door and open it. Outside is the long hallway with its rows of doors.

VII

As I close the door to 'Growth Room One' there is a faint tinkle at my feet, and I look down to see the key. I am surprised at how much smaller it is. It must have shrunk inside the lock and fallen out as I closed the door. I pick it up and try it in the lock and it's true - it doesn't fit at all now so I won't be able to lock the door. Experimentally, I try to open it again and it swings open easily. As I do so I notice that the sound of crying, which had got softer, gets louder again. I think of going back into the room and trying to get through the wall, but something tells me it will be a waste of time. So, reluctantly, I close the door and go to the next one along.

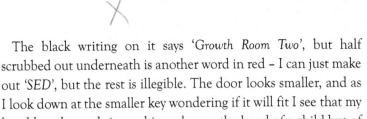

The black writing on it says 'Growth Room Two', but half scrubbed out underneath is another word in red – I can just make out 'SED', but the rest is illegible. The door looks smaller, and as I look down at the smaller key wondering if it will fit I see that my hand has changed size and is no longer the hand of a child but of a young adult. I put the key in the lock which is now at a sensible height for me, and it turns smoothly as though it has been well oiled. Silently the door opens on well-engineered hinges, and I go in half dreaming – half forgetting the crying that I am seeking.

I walk by saffron drapes on a carpet of silver fur. A huge painting of a lion fighting a tiger greets me on the opposite wall. Rending flesh. Who will win? The tiger ripping open the lion's belly or the lion throttling the tiger with his huge claws and mouth?

I turn away from this disturbing image to see a row of bottles on a polished table. A thought comes to me – insistent, compulsive:

'Drink and forget the pain, enjoy yourself. Go on, life's too short.'

I go over to the table and pour amber liquid into a crystal glass. As I raise it to my lips I notice a mirror on the wall behind the table. I see my face in it, not as I would like to see it, but a red face with bulging veins, broken capillaries – blood-shot eyes, stained teeth. The face of an alcoholic. I jump back, spilling my drink, and look down in horror as the liquid burns a hole in the silver fur. The glass falls from my hand and disintegrates into tiny fragments sending up a cloud of sparkling dust.

Frozen to the spot, I cautiously look around to see if anyone has noticed, but I am alone in this luxurious room. There's another full-length mirror further down the wall and I go to it to see if I look any different from the drunkard I so don't want to be. I see myself naked. A beautiful curvy body, luxuriant hair, young fresh face. The body of a flowering young woman. How gorgeous I am. How I just want to look and admire myself, turn this way and that to admire my lines. I turn and see behind me a table stocked with

stacked

69

all sorts of colourful clothing in soft expensive material. I would like to put it on. Try this or that outfit. Make myself feel better in all this lovely clothing. I deserve it after all. I've worked so hard. I pick up a long purple dress, the material is so soft, and yet it sparkles as though made of expensive gems. As I press it in front of my body and turn to see how it looks in the mirror, I hear the distant crying again. I drop the dress, distracted, remembering why I am here. I look down and see the dress writhing on the fur, its smooth surface gradually changing to scales. A darting tongue, two yellow eyes. I'm looking at a snake. I leap back involuntarily and knock the table over. As I look round I see all the colourful clothes begin to wriggle and writhe on the silver fur. I must escape from this room of snakes and acid, but it's become so big now that I can't see a way out.

Objects spring up into my vision, as though I am thinking them into existence. I seem to be in a large department store, and I'm very tired having walked around it for so long.

I see a large soft bed and the thought comes to me that I could just take a rest. I'm so tired, I just want to lie down on this bed and close my...

There's that crying again. I'm not going to go to sleep, I'm going to find the poor soul who is crying. I must find her, it's the most important thing in my life at this moment.

The room has regained its original shape again, the silver fur, the saffron drapes. But the painting has changed: the tiger lies dead beneath the victorious lion – its throat ripped open, and its glazed eyes staring at the door. The door! I must get out! Even as I start towards it I notice a movement in the corner of my eye, and there are the snakes coming to stop me, coming to poison me. I run for it and manage to get hold of the handle before a snake reaches me and bites my heel. The pain is unbelievable as I stagger out of the door and slam it, catching the snake in it and chopping its head off. After a moment of writhing the head turns into a piece of purple silk, just like the dress I wanted to try on, and even though I feel sick and giddy with the pain of the poisonous bite, I want to pick it up and feel it again. The crying is louder now and seems more urgent. I am caught between the twin desires of gratification and exploration. I can feel the poison in my veins working its way up to blur my sight and muddle my mind. I must move or I will never get away from this room. Painfully and slowly, with tremendous effort I reach for the key in the door and try to pull it out. It takes all my strength and as it comes out I see that it has gone rusty as if I had only just removed it in time to stop it rusting into the lock completely.

VIII

I turn and hobble down the hallway, the pain in my heel subsiding bit by bit as I get further away from that hellish room. The crying is still audible, indeed it seems to get louder as I reach the next door. The door is old and rough. More like a shed door, weathered and discoloured. The writing on it is scarcely legible: '*Leading to Growth Rooms ...*' The rest has disappeared, washed away by time. Instead of a neat lock in the door there is a rusty old padlock holding a hinged clasp, and I take the key and put it in the keyhole and try to turn it. It is stuck, rusted by age. And to my horror I see my hands have aged too. No longer youthful, they are gnarled and wrinkly. The hands of an old woman, the joints swollen with arthritis, the nails ridged and discoloured. Was it the poison from the snake? The pain has subsided now, although my heel still feels tender. I try the lock again in anguish and frustration. The key turns and then comes away in my hand, the end broken off. I feel tears of impotence in my eyes. Am I going to die of old age before I discover the crying child? Rage gives me strength as I tug at the clasp and it breaks away from the door

71

frame. I pull at the door on its rusty hinges and it bends back, one hinge breaking off. I squeeze through the gap and find myself in an old brick-lined corridor. It is very narrow and the mouldering walls are wet and slimy. Lurid green moss and small ferns grow out of the rotting brickwork, and the floor is slippery – half mud, half flagstone. Light comes from the end of the corridor, and as I hobble down it, the crying gets louder.

I reach the end and find old sacking hanging down making a makeshift door. Light filters through the strands of filthy cloth, and now I brush through them to see the room I have been trying to reach.

It is a Victorian classroom – rank upon rank of old-fashioned desks with benches attached. Battered and ink-stained, they have those lids that you can raise to find your books. No doubt the teacher would inspect them every day and mete out punishment for any untidiness. As I look to my right, I see the blackboard and the teacher's desk, complete with ruler no doubt used for rapping an unfortunate pupil's knuckles. The windows are high to prevent looking out, but the sun streams in enticingly, bringing thoughts of break-time freedom in the fields outside. The crying is coming from a lone figure right up the other end of the classroom, far away from the blackboard and shrouded in darkness – the corner that the sunlight never reaches.

I hobble down the aisle between the rows of desks and find the sobbing child sitting at her desk holding an old dipping pen poised above a stained inkwell. She is about twelve years old, and as she looks up I see myself in her tear-stained face.

"I c... I cah... I can't," she sobs. "I doe... I don't u... understand."

The lined exercise book in front of her is dotted here and there with tear stains, and there is a grubby thumb mark at the top corner where she has opened the book. Apart from that there is nothing on the page. It is the first page of her exercise book and she has written nothing at all. How long has she been here, crying with her hand poised above the inkwell? Stuck.

I gently grip her upper arms with my old wrinkled hands and try to look into her eyes.

"What is it? What is it you don't understand?"

She won't look at me but hangs her head, drooping over her exercise book.

"This." She thrusts her left arm in front of me pulling away from my hands, and there, in the half-light, I see the scars.

"W... why do I do it? I don't want to do it... b... but everything hurts." She gasps out the last word with such a force that it makes me jump. The sudden inexplicable fury. She is trapped in her pain, anguish, anger. I knew that once, but I buried it with time, and so lost sight of it, leading my life in what I thought was a happy positive way. Now this. I have to understand, I have to help her understand, or we will be stuck in this gloomy classroom for ever. The key. Where's the key? It broke, but I didn't let go of it. I must have dropped it when I reached out to the child. I look down at the dark stained wooden floor at my feet, and there it is, the rusty key with the end broken off. But even as I reach down to pick it up it changes, and I find I'm holding a rusty penknife. The blade is so rusty that it could never cut anything ever again.

"Where's your mother?" I ask.

"Gone. They've all gone and left me here. Alone."

"What are you trying to write?"

"She, she explained everything. Then I was to go away and write it down, but when I got here I couldn't remember it. I never understood her anyway." She was sobbing less now and the words came out more easily.

"Who is she?"

"The old woman with the 'O' mouth."

That was the woman who let me into the house. Was she a wise-woman or a witch?

"Perhaps you will never understand," I say gently. "Maybe you

73

just have to forgive yourself."

She turns to look me full in the face, her eyes dark with anger. "Then I would have to forgive everyone!" she shouts. "I can't do that. I won't, I won't!"

I step back, shocked by the sudden outburst - the change from grief to rage. "Why, what did they do?" I know the answer before she tells me.

"They took everything away. My home, my freedom, my toys, my trees, my mind. They made me who I am and I don't want to be me. I want to be... a boy." She says this last part quietly, and I can see her looking back in time, into her imagination, to the 'boy' that she would have liked to have been.

"Who are *they*?"

"I don't know. God but there is no God, all those people who made me what I am. Life, but I don't want life."

"What do you want?"

"Mummy, I want Mummy. But she's gone... The 'O' woman said I could find a Mummy inside me, but I can't." She bursts into a fresh spasm of sobbing, and I reach forward and hug her. I take her in my arms and give her all the love I have. It's the only way. She must have love in this love-starved place or she will never grow. We must leave here, I realise. She must come with me and we must find that room with the writing table, and we must write our story.

I take her hand and gently pull her away from the desk. Fear suddenly fills her face, her body goes rigid. "But I'll be...," she whispers.

"What will you be?"

"Lost."

"No, come with me. You will understand. I promise."

"Promise?" So many broken promises in her eyes.

I can't say it again so I just nod, and pull her down the aisle between the desks, past the ruler, past the blackboard which has 'I

MUST NOT HARM MYSELF' chalked on it in big blunt capitals, out into the damp corridor and down to the broken door.

IX

We make an odd couple, old and young. Both worn down with life. Standing in the hallway looking for the door into the writing room. It was the second door that I tried right back at the beginning of this strange journey, so I lead her down the hall towards the front door looking at the doors on my left. But nothing looks the same as I remembered it – no longer Victorian, it looks cold and modern. With a sick feeling I look at the grey featureless doors which now have no handles, just Yale locks. I have no key, just a rusty penknife. Break in. That's what we must do. I look at my companion holding my hand, and in her other hand is a credit card.

"My mummy's. I stole it when I ran away." She flinches, expecting me to be angry. But I'm not really listening. I'm thinking. Is this the house where I started? Or do I have to go back through all the horrors that I have experienced to find the writing room? Is this why it all looks so different? I look at the right-hand doors, and they have changed too. No locks, no handles, just those rectangular steel plates you push against to get the door to open on its spring. But I don't want that side, I want the locked side, so I lead us to the door on the left that I think must be the writing room. Remembering breaking in to my own home when locked out by a careless mother once, I take the credit card and slip it into the gap in the doorframe pushing the Yale lock back. I push the door open and we go in. Thieves.

I must have miscounted. We are back in the room with those horrible black shiny flowers. But there is a big difference: nearly all the plants lie dead round the walls. I can only see one plant still living and it is half hiding a door on the other side of the room.

Intrigued, I walk across the big room holding my girl's hand with a firm grip – I don't want her running away; is that for my sake or hers, I wonder? As we near the plant with its tendrils creeping up the wall, I see a label hanging from its upper branches: *'How Can I Trust Anyone Again?'*

Trust. Yes, that's what we are both looking for.

I need it to get across that floor in the writing room next door, and she needs it to start forgiving all the wrongs she feels have been done to her. Trust - the most wonderful thing to have in life. But always hanging around in dark corners there is the fear of betrayal. I can feel my companion tense up as we near the plant.

"So true," she whispers, already in the thrall of this herbal monster.

"Don't look at it. It will stop you getting to where you want. You will never escape," I say through gritted teeth.

I can already imagine the other plants round the wall beginning to grow roots again. All that work for nothing. I grip her hand more firmly and run at the door. The creeper's tentacles have gripped onto it, but I hit it with my shoulder with so much force that they break off with a shriek and the door opens on its spring, letting us through. It springs back firmly into place, leaving the memory of that horrible room behind us.

X

I pause to get my breath back and become aware of the smell of books. How I love that smell – the smell of adventure and discovery, mingled with that warm comforting scent of paper and cloth. We are safe here. We are in a private library. It is a large and elegant room with a long dark stained oak table in the middle. The scent of beeswax polish mingles with the deep strong smell of the books. At one end of the room there are tall French windows looking out onto a garden. I look up to the vaulted ceiling and the old painted beams, then back along the room to the large dark polished door at the other end guarded by two empty suits of armour that glint dully in the light from the windows. On each side the walls are lined with books, and as I look closer, I can see that some of the spines are coloured while the others are a dull grey. At this point my companion tugs me in the direction of the French windows – she wants to go into the garden and play in the sun. But I know we need to look at these books. They are our way through. She doesn't know this yet. She hasn't got the reading bug, but she soon will – and then this whole world will open up to her.

I take her to the end of the wall nearest to the windows and crouch down to look at the spines. The coloured ones stand out. *Winnie-the-Pooh*, *A Bear Called Paddington*, *The Wind in the Willows*, C.S. Lewis and Nigel Tranter make odd company, and I begin to realise that these books are ordered according to when I read them throughout my life. The coloured spines showing which ones I read, and the grey spines the ones I missed. I pull out *The House at Pooh Corner* and sit down with my companion to share the precious atmosphere and humour of A.A. Milne's wonderful world. But I can see that she's distracted. The outside pulls her, the sunny garden after all her imprisonment is too much of a temptation. So I let her go, and she opens the French windows and walks out onto a fresh green lawn. The scent of old roses comes into the library, and I'm almost tempted to follow her and leave my books. But I am so fascinated to see my progression from child to adolescent to young adult. Books about animals, both real and fictional, seem to grab me early on. Then the *Lord of the Rings* period. But getting out of that, and feeling a bit lonely as not many girls that I knew read Tolkien, I launched myself into the classics. Almost as if I had to prove something. But I loved them: Greek, Roman, Italian, German, Russian, French. All in translation of course – I was no good at foreign languages. I read so much. How much did I understand? I wonder now. Then I discovered Hardy and his grief-driven stories of countryside and old England. No grey spines in that area. *Jude the Obscure* affected me so much in my twenties. God knows why, I must have been naturally depressed. Dickens – a few grey spines here, and I begin to realise that as I get older I become less and less capable of reading long tracts of description. I am hungry for plot. Hesse seems to satisfy this – his writing so succinct. Wonderful short novels so clear and to the point. But I have got a long way round the room, and realise that I have read comparatively little in my thirties.

My thirties? But I'm an old woman now. Where are all the later books in my life? This library is not showing me anything past the most recent novels that I read in my thirties. Interestingly, they are all contemporary. McCall Smith, Atkinson, Gaiman, Trapido, Winterson. Good quality writing but easy to read compared to the old classics. So that's it. The books I will read in later life have not been written yet, so of course I can't see them on the shelves. I look around, searching for more clues of what is to come, and the sunlight catches a grey spine with red writing on the back. I cross over to look more closely: *Crime and Punishment*, the book I tried to read three times. I never managed to get past the mare being flogged to death. It was all too cruel, I couldn't live with it. As I look round I realise there are an awful lot of grey spines with coloured lettering – books I started but never finished. And they get more and more numerous as I get older. Frustrating, those worlds that I couldn't get into. Treasures promised but never revealed to me.

I look out into the garden, suddenly alert – waking from my world of books. I have no idea how much time has passed, but the girl is nowhere to be seen. I go to the open French windows and look down the garden. No sign of her. I begin to feel panic – I just know we need to do the rest of this journey together. I try to run but am too old and stiff, so I totter as fast as I can down the long lawn to the trees. I call my name out "Mel, Mel!" my voice sounds strange after all this silence. Muffled by the garden world, oddly loud to my own ears but getting lost in all this green space. I round a bend between the trees, and there below me is a lake with a tiny island in the middle. Lawns border both sides of it, but all is hemmed in by a forest. If she has gone in there I will never find her. I go down to the lake half expecting to find her there, and as I reach it I see a ride between the trees leading off to the right. There is something familiar about this place, and as I turn down the ride, there in front of me are the fallen elms. I must be coming to them from the other side, and I see that they block the ride completely. As I get closer I see a small figure scrambling over the fallen trunks. It's her and I call. She turns and looks at me, but there is something taking her interest on the other side of the elms. As I get closer, to my horror, I see the boy with the mask. She is drawn towards him, attracted by his strange charm. He is holding a knife. I have a knife too, but mine is useless and rusty.

"No!" I shout, but my voice is swallowed up in this world. I know what will happen if she takes that knife. I must stop her – I throw my rusty penknife at the fallen trees in frustration. What on earth can I offer her that will distract her from this destructive boy? As I stumble towards the great fallen boles, something small and red catches my eye, and there on the ground by the first elm lies a ball. I pick it up and it fits in my hand as though it wants to be there. It has writing on it 'Catch me', in black and gold.

An instinct makes me shout "Catch!" to the girl, as she nears the other side of the fallen elms. She turns and I throw the ball to her. By some strange miracle she catches it. I see the amazement in her face – she didn't expect to catch that ball. She looks back at me with a smile of pure joy, and for the first time I get a glimpse of the happy girl that lived in a secure and loving home. She throws it back to me and it is my turn to be surprised. It seems to home in on my hand and I cannot help but catch it. I look up to see her scrambling back across the trunks towards me, the deathly boy forgotten in our game of catch. We need this, this game of connection, and I throw the ball back to her. She catches it with one hand as she balances on a log, and she makes her way back to me with an easy grace that belies her long incarceration in that gloomy classroom. How long was she there? Most of my life, I suspect.

We play catch all the way back up to the lake, and stop there to look at our reflections in the still waters. One old, one young, but the same. Connected by a ball, by a game, by fun. We turn to each other and laugh, and we play with our ball as the sun goes down behind the trees. Gradually we make our way up to the house in the dusk. We will have to stop soon, and it will be hard to go back into the house and on with our journey. I am worried that I will lose the girl at the last minute, and that she will be stuck here forever with the constant threat of the boy. But as we near the house, a change comes over the ball. It gets heavier, and begins to glow. She has it in her hand now, and she looks down, marvelling at this beautiful thing. She is holding a golden globe. 'A *light to guide us home*' comes into my mind. It must have come into hers as well, because she makes straight for the French windows and leads the way into the library, lighting it up with the globe in her hand. We walk down the long dark room, past the polished table with the light of our globe reflecting on it, to the door at the other end, and we open it.

XI

The golden globe slips from her fingers and we are plunged into darkness. At first I can see nothing, then as my eyes become accustomed to the dark, I see ashes, ashes everywhere. My feet are walking on soft ash, and I look down at shades of black and grey wondering why this makes me so sad. No, I don't want to be here.

I turn to find the door but all I can see in the dim light is burnt peeling wallpaper. A charred wedding photo still hanging on the wall where the door used to be. I try to make out the couple in the picture – they are very familiar. It's all horribly familiar. Then I hear her crying, heart-rending sobs, and I realise we are in the burnt-out ruins of our old home. She stands still, crying, keening, for her lost family, her lost home. She falls to her knees and starts rummaging in the ashes as though she will find something – bring something back. But there is no return, no bringing back. All those people, all that love. Gone.

We must get through this ruin. Grief hits me in a huge wave, and I can't move for the ache inside my body. Slowly my knees give way and I join the stricken girl on the floor feeling through the ashes for something. Searching to find our lost world. But it is useless, useless, useless.

Then my hand comes across a small hard object. A ring. I carefully pick it out of the ashes, blowing away the grey dust from it. It is my auntie Doris's wedding ring. I know it. She used to take it off when she was baking, and sometimes she would sit me on her knee and let me try it on – large and loose on my little-child finger.

I can hear her say, "One day you'll be married, and you can wear a ring like this. Won't that be lovely."

I put it on my bare ring finger now and it fits. A slim simple band of gold. A piece of her, a bit of the past to carry with me. I take the girl's hands and pull her gently to her feet. We have to get through this, we can't search through the ashes for ever. My auntie's ring has given me strength – she was a strong woman.

Was.

I feel grief rising in my throat again.

Walk.

We must walk through this and bear the sadness.

The smoke-blackened walls hold the darkness in, as we shuffle along the old ruined· hallway. Memories come back to me, of family feasts held here at Christmas or other special occasions. The staircase at the end is gone. Just a pile of charred wood and ashes. Their way out that they never had a chance to use. We turn and take a narrow corridor to the right. We should go under the stairs and into the servants' quarters at this point, but that has all burnt away, and all I can see is an old blackened toilet – the Bakelite seat melted into a bizarre shape in the cracked and blackened bowl. Light floods in from the bathroom window next door, and the bath is full of plaster and burnt lathes. We walk down what used to be a corridor, past the larder to the dining room and a shock greets me here. The back end wall of the house has fallen out and I am looking straight down into the courtyard twenty feet below. These memories of a past world that I thought I'd long forgotten are broken into by this devastation. I can see the floor is likely to give way if we go any further so I grab her hand and pull her back down the corridor to the relative safety of the hall. I look up to see the moon shining through a huge hole in the roof two floors above us, and in the pool of light it sends down onto the floor, I see a little arm. The girl's on it quick as a flash, and pulls a blackened doll out of the ashes. My doll. The doll that kept me company when I was alone because the boys went off and did boy things. She hugs it to herself – I want to hug it too but I am old now and the memory will have to do. Instead I turn and look into what was once our sitting room where we sat round the fire chatting and playing games. It looks much smaller than I expected. So dark in there – just a pile of burnt rubble. The old sofa would have gone up like a firelighter, but there are still a couple of rusty springs sticking out of the ashes – all that remains of a comfortable family resting place. I look for the Uccello, it has fallen off the wall, the half-burnt frame and shattered glass revealing the brave nobleman still brandishing his useless baton, his magnificent headdress blackened by fire. One French window remains, the other has burnt out leaving a pile of broken glass for us to step through.

We make our way gingerly into the garden, careful to avoid cutting our bare feet. The gravel of the path feels hard and prickly after all that soft ash, and in the moonlight we see our once beautiful garden transformed into a jungle of weeds. Cow parsley grows six feet high. There are brambles and nettles everywhere, and the grass that remains has grown into rough browning hummocks. No sign of the lovely flat lawn where we played croquet with an old battered set handed down from god-knows-where. As I peer into the mass of foliage I can just make out a rusty hoop and a rotten mallet. The boys were always being told off for forgetting to put the croquet things away – they pretended the mallets were guns in their games round the garden. I hold the girl's hand and we stand there in the silver light, lost in our memories.

A movement catches my eye. There is some creature out there in the bushes that border the lawn-that-was. A flash of white, the crack of a broken twig. We are both attracted towards the movement, and the moonlight picks out a narrow track between the nettles and brambles. We go in single file, the girl leading, and I can feel her fear – this garden was always full of ghosts at night. The path takes us to the bushes, and we enter a tunnel of rhododendrons grown so high we can easily make our way through without stooping. We see a flash of white at the end of the tunnel, and it spurs us on. We come out into the old orchard. Pear and apple trees surround us and suddenly we are hungry.

We each pick a ripe-looking apple from the biggest tree right in the middle of the orchard, and as we eat we change. I feel better, younger. The pain in my heel, which I have been stoically ignoring, goes, and a warm feeling fills my limbs. I look at the girl and she has grown slightly taller. She has lost that sad look that dogged her pretty features, and has a look of contentedness that is unusual in a girl in her early teens. The sadness of our lost home is seeping away. Even the orchard is looking tidier and less neglected, and for the first time I notice a green wooden door set into the fence on the other side of the orchard. There is no sign now of the creature that led us here, but the door beckons, and we both walk through the trees as though pulled by an invisible thread.

XII

The door has a rounded top which fits neatly into a hoop of climbing roses. The latch is freshly painted black and clicks in a satisfying way as I press my thumb on it. It opens easily, and we find ourselves in a yard outside a rambling Victorian house. I am sure this is the house I started in, but I'm just viewing it from the back. It has the same arched windows and eccentric architectural features. There is a driveway round the side which might take us to the front, but something makes me unwilling to meet the 'O' woman again. Anyway my companion has already run to the back door and disappeared inside. She leaves the green door ajar and I wander in; the mixed smells of overcooked cabbage and polish greet me.

School!

A long dark corridor with polished wooden floor and painted brick walls – two-tone cream and red leads me into the bowels of the house. School. The last place I want to be, and for her a terrible place that I have just freed her from. If she gets back into that classroom she could be stuck there forever. I see her turn right at the end of the corridor and I run after her, my limbs younger and more willing now. As I get to the end I am just in time to see her turn right again a shorter distance ahead. I am catching up with her. She turns right again, and again. We must be going round in a circle. Finally I catch up with her. We have ended up in a tall dark room, a bit like a prison cell. The two-tone paint is still on the walls. Institutional. There is a bit of light coming from a window set high up in the wall. This room makes me feel very claustrophobic and I turn to go back out the way we came in. I make a grab at the girl's hand but she's too fast for me and has run to a door on the other side of the room and disappeared again.

More cautiously this time, I follow her and almost stumble up stone steps spiralling up into the dark. I hear her footsteps up ahead but can see nothing. It is pitch black now and I'm using my hands to guide me, feeling the steps in front of me – almost going up on all fours. I nearly collide with her in the dark – she has stopped in front of me. She is grunting with effort as she pushes up against something above her head. I get alongside her and reach up to feel wooden boards. A trapdoor?

We both push upwards and our combined efforts cause the boards to move upwards with a reluctant creak. Light and warmth stream down on us and we push the trapdoor as far as it will go, and peer up over the rim into what appears to be a large comfortable old room. We climb up and out onto an old red Persian rug which covers the floor. At the other end is a cheerful log fire in a large inglenook fireplace. A very comfortable sofa is set at an angle to the fireplace, and beyond it a corridor leads into darkness again. I just want to sit down on the sofa and rest. I feel an overpowering urge to just go to sleep in this warm comforting room. Journey's end. Job done. No more struggle. No more pain. The temptation is too great. I sit down on the sofa and feel myself nodding off.

I jerk awake. Where is the girl? What am I doing? I want to go back to the writing room. I haven't finished. I don't want to finish here. I want to live. I struggle up off the sofa, it feels as if a magnetic force is keeping me there. With a huge effort I get to my feet and stagger out of the room. Another dark spiral staircase greets me at the end of the corridor and I climb up into the darkness again.

It's not long before I find her pushing up against yet another trapdoor. This one is much heavier, and we need all her growing strength and my increasingly youthful body to make it budge. As we push hard, it begins to move, sending bits of damp soil down onto the steps and onto our arms. The trapdoor has evidently been covered in earth, and when we eventually manage to heave it open, more soil falls on us and into our eyes and hair.

As we clamber up and out onto the muddy floor, I realise that I've been here before. It's not so dark as it was. The roots have gone and I can hear the sea. We could just walk out to the beach. I feel a wrench inside me – I want to go to that paradise, and swim in the warm bay, but also I feel the urgent need to get to that writing room before I leave the house. Once again my companion makes my decision for me and continues on up the steps. I follow her, and we come into the middle of the Unforgiven room.

All the plants are dead. They lie in rotting piles around the walls. The floor is slimy with their rancid sap, and the stench is overpowering. The girl wants to escape up the spiral staircase, but I grab hold of her hand and pull her with me, half sliding across the slippery floor. We must get to the door. We must not fall over – I can feel the acidity of this sludge eating into my feet. I wouldn't like this all over me. I retch, and am almost sick, as I stagger across to the door. How could I ever have been attracted to this room? We pull on the door and it opens towards us, pushing a wave of nauseating sludge over our feet and back into the room. We are out.

The hall has regained its original Victorian appearance. Locked doors opposite us and no need to use a key, or even a credit card, on this side. I look down at my feet and am dismayed to see red raw blisters developing where the skin is visible beneath the green slime. There must be a bathroom. Something tells me I must wash my feet before attempting the writing room again. My poor feet are beginning to itch and sting as I hobble down the hall looking for a sign. We reach the grand stairs at the end, and I gaze up wondering if they really go on into infinity. The girl tugs at me and points down a short corridor on our right to a small door with the word 'Bathroom' painted in dark green on it.

XIII

We enter the bathroom cautiously. A large white bath on legs
is in the centre of the room. Towels are hung on golden painted
chairs around the bath, and a small marble table is set with lotions
and soaps. The bath already has clean water in it and we step
in holding hands to support each other. The water is warm, and
although it stings to start with, it soon soothes our poor blistered
feet. The water smells sweet and aromatic, taking away the rancid
smell of decay. We both perch on the edge of the bath and I reach
for some soap to wash my companion's feet. It's a beautiful thing
to do, and I feel her relax as I massage and soothe her blistered
soles. I stoop down to wash my own feet, but she tugs at my
arm and takes the soap from me to do it for me. What a blissful
sensation after all that walking on my bare feet, and then being
infected by the acidic sap of bitterness. She soothes it all away with
her young hands, and I feel so clean and warm.

We both help each other out of the bath, and dry our feet with
soft white towels. I try some lotion from a purple bottle on one
foot, and feel the energy rush up through my body. I carry on
rubbing it into the other foot and then onto hers. As I stand
up I feel inches taller, and I take her hand and walk out of the
bathroom and up the hall, carefully avoiding the puddles of green
bile that we left on the way down.

As we near the end of the hall, I can hear the murmur of voices.
It is coming from the room that I have wanted to get back to for
so long. The writing room. It sounds like the large round room
is full of people, and the tone of their voices has a gentle quality
– almost reverential, as though the 'other' in person is in that
room. We pause in front of the door, reluctant to go in and spoil
the joy of the gathering. I feel suddenly shy, wondering what all

these people will make of us - two strays lost in this mysterious world. We gently open the door and look in. A hush falls, and at first I can't see any people. The table is in the middle of the room on a little platform. The blue light reflects on the circular wall. Then I look down and see... hands. The floor which was once so treacherous is now made up of hands. Palms upwards, they make a human carpet to the centre of the room. We stand on the lip, unsure what to do. The hands move slightly. There are people down there beneath those hands. People who will let us walk on their outstretched hands to get to the writing table. As we pause uncertainly, a murmur starts up.

> "Come on, come in,
> Walk on our hands and we'll support you,
> Walk on our palms and we'll support you,
> Soles on our palms and we'll support you,
> Come on, come in."

And we take our first step off the lip and onto the crowd of hands.

The feel of having my feet held up by these strong hands is strange, ticklish and sensuous. As we step slowly and carefully, each hand we step onto grips each foot gently to support us so we don't stagger or fall on this bizarre surface. I have a vision of atoms, and how curious it is that we don't fall through the gaps between them as we walk on a floor. We trust them without even thinking about it. These hands are huge atoms, and we must trust them. In fact this is all about trust. All those people below us are holding us up, and this is how it is.

Trust.

It feels like a long way to the table in the middle of the room. Our progress is slow and careful - each step is important. It doesn't just involve us, but also each person who holds us up as we go past.

"Come on, come in."

I hear their chant inside my head, regular and rhythmic. Very stabilising and encouraging, as it comes from beneath me, from the people who are holding me up. But it's inside my head at the same time, as if I'm making it happen. A regular breath-step music, that swells as we get to the middle of the room and then subsides with a gentle sigh as we reach the little platform with the writing table on it.

Silence. Silence as we sit down on the two chairs provided and pull them up to the table. Silence as we start to write. We write what is in our minds – our stories, and once we start it feels like we will never stop. I glance at my companion. She has a determined look on her face. Concentrated. Not the expression of total despair that she had when she was stuck in the classroom. She writes smoothly and fluently, pausing every now and then to consider the next word or phrase.

I return to my writing and find the words forming in my mind like a flowing river. Ideas I never knew I had, places I'd never seen, people I'd never met. They all come out onto the page, ready formed and real. A story to hold me in its arms, and carry me on through life. An endless undercurrent forming and flowing beneath my surface. Always there, always available, always trustworthy. I write of mysteries, of ideas that were once fleeting shadows in my mind. Now they return fully formed to amaze me with their completeness. Connections, thoughts of wisdom, joy and sadness all flow from my pen, and I cover sheet after sheet. No-one is looking over my shoulder, no-one is telling me when to stop.

I have no idea how long I have been here, writing to save my life – to tell my life. But I look up and see that my companion has stopped and is looking at me expectantly. I have come to an end, for now, so I reluctantly get up and look round the room. The hands, the people, have vanished. And in their place is the old beautiful oak floor, shining with a blue light. I hear the sea again and I am reminded of a place, a beach, a forest. The smell of pines and salt lure me and I must go.

I take the girl's hand and we walk across the smooth wooden floor leaving our writings behind us. We may find them another day, but now it is time to leave. No threat of crumbling floor now. We are held above a vast chasm, and this we know. But we will not fall, the floor will not give way. It will carry us to the edge, to the door and out to the hall with all its doors and mysteries. As we reach the door there is a faint murmur, a goodbye, and we leave replenished, hopeful and ready for whatever will come next. We go down the hallway to the front door and leave the house. There is no 'O' woman there to say goodbye. She has gone, taking so much grief and trouble with her.

XIV

We walk up the sandy slope away from the house, our eyes fixed on the trees and the path through them that will take us to the sea. It is night again and the moon is still full. It lights our path with silver. The sand beneath our feet makes no sound, and we seem to glide down a beam of light to our destination. We turn a corner and I notice that the roots of trees have grown above ground in certain places. I don't remember this coming the other way, we will have to go carefully now or we will trip. My companion stumbles and stubs her toe. With a howl she sits down abruptly and clutches her injured foot, rocking backwards and forwards with the pain. I sit down beside her and put my arms round her, to give her comfort. But as I do so, the moon goes behind a cloud and it goes completely dark.

I shiver with the sudden cold. I don't like being with all these roots in the dark. A wind gets up, and it gets even colder. We hug

90

each other in the darkness, frightened now. I was so sure that we would get down to the beach easily, and finish our journey.

But now we are stuck in the dark surrounded by roots, the memories of resentments I thought we had left behind. I reach out blindly and touch a root. I feel its fine bristly hairs. It has lost its way coming above ground, only to be mauled and broken by trampling feet. Useless. And I feel sorry for it. It is frightened, haunted. Not me. I am going to the beach, and I have no intention of getting stuck here. I take her hand in the darkness and get up carefully. Cautiously, we inch our way along the path, feeling each root with our feet and stepping over it. There is a moment when we come across a root that is knee high and I wonder if we have left the path, but we get over it and the smooth sand under my feet tells me we are still going in the right direction. It takes time and patience to get along this last bit of the path to the beach, but I am encouraged by the smell of the sea blown onto our faces by the wind, and by the sound of the surf swelling and receding in a natural lulling rhythm.

This lullaby of nature brings us home, and as the path seems to broaden on both sides, the moon comes out and we see the beach looking almost circular as it curves round the bay. We walk up out of the forest, and onto the sandy bank at the highest part of the beach. From there we can see the dim shapes of islands across the water, and distant mountains shrouded in mist.

But now we begin to dance on this sand beneath a diamond sky, and I hold the hand of my younger self, looking straight into her eyes, my other hand waving free. We circle slowly to start with, finding a rhythm in our bodies that is in time with the surf. The gentle pulse pulls us round and round, and with each circle some more grief falls away. We dance on in bliss, gradually getting faster and faster. We feel light, as though we are flying, and we start to spin, getting so fast that we become a blur. Two bodies no longer separate, but one in this crazy dance. Then we fall over, laughing, and lie back on the soft sand looking up at the moon.

After my head has stopped spinning I reach out to touch my companion, but there is no-one there. I ease myself up on my elbow to look for her, but she is gone. That girl that was me, caught in a dark classroom, has joined me now. And I am whole. I scan the beach to make sure, but there is no sign of my girl-self. Something catches my eye at the high end of the beach. It looks like a rucksack, and I slowly get up to investigate. I still feel a bit dizzy, and wobble my way up to have a look. There is something in the rucksack, and as I get closer I see a little face. Eyes closed. It is a baby, fast asleep in a back carrier, propped up facing the sea. I reach out to touch it, but my hand goes straight through it. I long to pick it up – to cuddle it, but I can't. It is a ghost. My baby that I never had, and I long for it now. My baby. Is this where I go next? To create new life? To give my body to another soul, and to nurture it? Will that ever be possible again?

I turn to the sea, and I feel its call. It is time to go now, 'deep beneath the waves'. The sea is warm and inviting. I walk slowly into the gentle ripples. It comes up to my knees, then up to my waist. I walk out further and further until it reaches my shoulders. Then it goes over my head and I am going down into this blue sea-world. The sound of water is in my ears, everything else is muted. But still I can see. Clear light and curving currents. I don't need to breathe, everything is slowing down. This warm sea gives a gentle resistance to every movement I make. I am gliding in slow motion in this wide empty sea. Blue surrounds me, and water fills my ears, my nose and my mouth. It doesn't matter, I'm finding my destination, my end. My infinity.

Then I look down, and I am at the top of the stairs in the Dreamhouse. Strangely, I am underwater but over air. I can see people walking about. Little dots moving up and down the hallway, going in and out of rooms. Rooms that I never went in, and I wonder what they might be about. Guilt? Obsession? Need

92

to be admired? Gratitude? Oh yes, I feel grateful. Full of gratitude to my dead family, and to all those people who took my weight on their hands, and let me write my story. But the other rooms? Have I got past them? Do I need to visit them some time in the future? Am I quite finished? I shudder suddenly, and the water feels cold. In the distance above me, I can hear a voice saying something about catching. Catching what? Fish?

There it is again, "Catch her." But I'm not a fish, and I need to breathe. I look up and begin to panic. I can see light above me. Air. I need to swim up. My lungs are bursting. I can't breathe. I struggle up through the weight of water, arms and legs flailing desperately in my attempt to reach the surface before I drown. The light gets closer, the voices become clearer. I hear his voice. The man I love. He is weeping now, "I should have caught her." He sounds heartbroken as I reach the surface. It feels like I am driven up by the buoyancy of the water and I almost jump up in bed, eyes wide open, gasping for breath.

They all look at me in amazement. The doctor, the nurse, Mark, and James - tears streaming down his face. I am sitting up in bed, fully conscious, and they are staring at me.

"I thought she'd gone." James's voice hoarse with emotion.

"Eem ell yeet," bloody hell, my voice still doesn't work. How can I tell them I'm alright? I smile, and that seems to work. There is joy, relief, concern all mixed up in their expressions. I am made of alabaster. Will no-one touch me? I won't disintegrate, I'm me. I'm whole. Then gentle hands push me back down into the pillows. Doctors and nurses teem round me like small fish round a stranded whale. I feel stranded now, here in bed. Unable to do anything but smile, and let them do their tests and make me safe.

Then they go and I feel him take my hand. There he is. My reason for coming back. He called me up from the sea, and I heard his call and swam to him. He is my risk. Another person. Another world. Someone else to consider, to worry about, to cause me grief. But to love. It overwhelms me and I feel the warmth in my body as I take his hand in both of mine.

" I yuvooh," I murmur.

The Party

Chapter 12

I drink a cup of tea. It is made with love, with care. The flavour is full, chocolaty, and the colour is just right – not too dark, but not insipid and pointless. A little steam comes off the surface; I feel it go up my nose and provide a warmth in the cool early-morning air.

I am in a garden. Not the never-ending garden of my dreams, but a well-tended garden at the back of James's house. He had kept his garden a secret from me till I came to live with him. Now I live in his garden. At least as much as I can. My world is small at the moment. Limited to a wheelchair, and the love of another person who wheels me around and looks after me. It is a small world, but it is beautiful. I can see so much from my wheelchair. Out here in his garden I can watch a butterfly make its journey of nectar-gathering and doing other mysterious things that I don't understand. But I can fly with it in my imagination as it roves round the flowers and shrubs in James's garden. Until it goes over the fence and disappears, maybe to fly thousands of miles. My mind goes with it for a while, imagining its wondrous journey until something else takes my attention.

But this morning at six o'clock I am listening as I sip my tea. Birdsong. Another mystery. What are they doing? Some of it is very repetitive. The wren declaring its territory – its shrill voice seems powerful for such a small creature, as it shouts at the other birds. But what is the blackbird up to? Its song ranges from some typical blackbird phrases into long improvisations. Maybe it is just joy, but I feel it could be language. Communication. After all, blackbirds are the main communicators in the garden, warning the others of a potential predator with their insistent cry.

And here's a predator now. An early morning cat out for a stroll. It's Tess. And she's come to see me. Small, whitish, she has an exquisite face with lovely almond eyes. She looks at me, as usual, with an expression of faint astonishment. I don't know what her game is but she will hang around watching me as if I were something really interesting, but she won't let me touch her. I have tried, but I am slow and clumsy and she always darts back out of my reach. Still, she's company, and we talk with our eyes until it is her breakfast time. Then she is off and disappears into the mysterious house next door. And that's that.

It is Saturday today and James isn't working, so we can have the day together. On Monday I am going to a new clinic to have physio, and to try and take that first step again. I am dreading it. I know I need to, that I don't want to be in a wheelchair for the rest of my life, but just for now I enjoy the dependence. Snuggled up in my chair watching the world in minute detail. I never saw it this way when I could move about at will. Always restless, something to do. Driven.

So, today is Saturday, and James's friends will come round for a nibbles party at six. I look forward to that. It's entertaining watching people trying to work out what I'm saying in the secure knowledge that James will translate if we get stuck. Some people are really good at deciphering my mumbles and odd vowels. They must be good at foreign languages – or at least my foreign language. Others, perfectly intelligent, are completely baffled by the simplest clearest word.

The door creaks behind me and I hear James's footsteps. He puts his arm on my shoulder and kisses the top of my head.

"Would you like another cuppa?" He sees my mug is still half full. I'd forgotten to drink while I was thinking.

"Are you alright? Your tea's gone cold," he looks at me with concern. I've failed the tea test. Something must be wrong.

"Oobs edot. Sun, beds," I gesture round the garden, "waz indin."

James translates back to me to make sure he's understood. "Oh, you forgot. You were thinking, enjoying the sun and appreciating my flower beds."

I laugh, "Beds nod beds!" I make a flapping motion with my hands to indicate birds. "Sinnin."

James smiles, presses my hands and picks up my mug to replenish it with more gorgeous tea. He really is the most wonderful man, and tea maker. I wish I could stop him from worrying so much. Still, the language thing is vexing. More than that, it's a huge barrier. At the moment I have lost essential sounds like 'err', 'oar', 'k', 'g', 'ing', 'p'. Those are the worst. You'd be surprised how many words have the 'oar' sound in them. Here am I hearing the words in my head and coming out with such garbled results. It's very frustrating. I do wonder what it must be like to be born with this impediment. Never having been able to easily say what you want. Having to learn every word from scratch. I knew a little girl once, who could read perfectly well, and obviously understood complicated conversation. She had a big vocabulary inside her head but had to painstakingly work out how to say each word with huge effort. What a massive task. I really respect her now. At least I have spoken clearly in the past, so I know it can be done again. Hopefully. That's one thing I really look forward to – speech therapy. The gateway to connecting my world to other people's.

James comes back with another mug of steaming tea. He puts it on the little garden table beside me and draws up a battered old wooden chair to sit by me and enjoy the garden, which is now full of early morning sunlight.

In some ways, talking to James seems to be unnecessary. He reads my mind so well, as I read his. But we both know that the more I talk the better, and he is so able to understand and help.

I pick up my mug, revelling in my improved ability to hold and handle it safely. Fine motor skills coming along nicely. There's no accounting for the ever-mending neurological pathways in the brain. Some less experienced medics will put people into boxes, but a neurologist worth his salt will know these boxes don't exist. Every person is different, and convenient though boxes might be, they generally get in the way.

These mugs that James has are made of bone china, with lovely pictures of rural scenes painted under the fine glaze. He insists on drinking tea out of bone china, and I think he is right. There is something very different about the feeling, and the way food and drink feels is as important as its taste. So when I say 'cup of tea', I generally mean 'mug'. In fact it's a rare thing to drink tea out of a cup and saucer these days, and I doubt my fine motor skills would be up to it. Wobble, wobble, clunk, clunk, and half of the tea would be already tepid in the saucer.

I drink the freshly poured tea and savour the rich flavour of the second cup – deeper and more chocolaty than the first. Mmmmh.

Chapter 13

He has adapted his house for me. Conveniently, there is a spare room downstairs that I was able to move in to. James brought my stuff from the pub where it was stored for the months I was in hospital. My room is at the back of the house well away from his consulting room at the front. Clients can come and go without my hearing or seeing them. So they can feel safe and undistracted, and I can get on with my life unimpeded. The loo downstairs has been adapted with bars to hold on to, so I can get from my wheelchair onto the toilet without too much effort. This recently found freedom is really special for me. Surprising how much better life is when you can at least pee and poo in private. He has put in a sit-down shower, no expense spared – and these things are expensive, believe me. It was all done so quickly and painlessly. I think he must have some reserves of money, and I wonder if it is the insurance pay-out after his wife's accident. He doesn't talk about it, and I'm afraid to ask – it would seem so ungrateful.

Another area we don't go into is sex. I long to make love. A big part of me wants to have his baby. But I am not ready physically. The closest we get is the loving way he helps me in and out of the shower – the way he helps me dry myself, and helps me with my clothes. He likes my body, I know it. And I probably turn him on, but he does the restraint thing very well. Maybe we will make love soon. I hope so. But will I ever be able to have a baby? That remains to be seen.

He does have great hands. He massages my lower back, which gets stiff and sore from being in that chair all day. I do like that. A recompense for all the discomfort. He's strong. He holds me. He is my man, and – oh god, that's scary – I need him, can't live without him. Suppose he changes his mind. Turns away from me. Blocks me out.

So here I am in my bedroom getting ready for the party – I push that fear away and concentrate on trying to get my earrings in. This is quite a challenge, getting my fingers to make such fine movements. I spike my neck. Have I drawn blood? I feel with my fingers where the hurt is. Now I think I might know what it's like being a man cutting himself shaving. But no, no blood. Try again. Left hand hold earlobe to guide right hand in with hook of earring. My right hand shakes uncontrollably for a moment. I feel tears in my eyes. Self-pity. Frustration. I'm going to give up.

Then I remember my auntie Doris and her words of encouragement. Sitting on her knee, trying on her ring. I look down at my right hand holding the earring, and there is her ring. The memory of her on my ring finger.

Right. That's better. Start again. A steadiness takes my hand, as though it were being guided, and I get the hook up to my left ear. Just one fine movement and it will be in. But I'm thinking about it too much – my left arm's aching and I'm holding my earlobe too hard. I drop my hands to my lap. Exhausted. I so wanted to surprise him. To look beautiful for him without having to call on him for help.

Come on, come on. Concentrate.

Then through the window I hear the blackbird. Its song is different this evening. More complex. Hugely varied, with swirls and whirls of bubbling sound. And then clear notes followed by one of its more recognisable patterns. Then off on a musical tangent again. Unexpected phrases. I am enthralled. My hands are moving up to my ear again. The hook of the earring goes through the tiny hole in my flesh, and one pretty silver earring is in place.

How did I do that? Automatically, that's how. I got distracted, stopped thinking, and my brain took over – following old familiar patterns. Of course, I never thought about how I put my earrings in. I just did it. Trusted in my reflexes, my fingers knowing where they were in space. When you start thinking about how you do these simple things, they become impossibly complex.

Now try the other ear. The more difficult one. I'm right handed so using my left hand will be... impossible? No. Don't think, just do. But that's easier said than done. How do you stop yourself from thinking? I was distracted by the blackbird before, but I didn't know it. This time my brain is alert, confusing my reflexes. Not trusting them.

I look in the mirror. Yes, I am very pretty. I'm looking into big sparkling blue eyes. Nice cheekbones, good skin. How lucky to have that. As I look, I smile and it lights up my whole face and I become beautiful, not just pretty. As I watch my spreading smile, I feel my hands moving in a familiar pattern and my earring is hooking into my right ear. My hand jerks at the last moment, and the earring's hook pulls in my earlobe causing me a sharp pain. But through the mist of tears in my eyes I can see my two earrings in place, glinting in the frame of my long brown hair. True, as the mist clears, I notice the red blotches on my poor lobes. The right one still stinging. But I've done it, and though I feel tired from my exertions, I am elated too. Another little victory, and as though on cue James knocks on my door.

I turn as he comes in, and I see surprise on his face, mixed with a sort of disappointment that I can't understand.

"You got them in yourself, but... " He trails off, and I notice him put his hand behind his back. Then he registers what I've done, and the look on his face makes it all worth it.

"I... I got you these." He brings his hand out from behind his back and shows me a little black box. He's about to open it for me, but I want to do it. It's fiddly for my clumsy challenged fingers, but I can do it. I reach my hand out and he places the box in it and stands back to watch me. My hands shake as I try to open it, and they suddenly jerk as it comes open, spilling the contents onto the floor in front of me.

103

I look down and two diamonds shine up at me. "Yey're booful," I gasp, staring at them and then at him. And I wonder at what possessed him to buy me two expensive diamond studs after all the other things he has done for me. I see something in his eyes – something else there, and I wonder if he'd bought them for his wife, Alice, as he kneels down and picks them up tenderly.

"I was going to put them in for you, but you… No, you should keep those in, you got them in." He is happy for my victory now – a big moment in my recovery. "We can try them in later."

It's awkward, I want to ask, 'Were they for her?' but it seems so ungrateful. Alice is dead. Have I taken her place? I don't want to, I just want him to love me for my sake. I reach out and take his hand, and I feel a surge of electricity pass between us. I've never held a hand that felt like this – so natural, so at home. I want to make love to him there and then – me in a wheelchair, him on his knees. He comes close and we kiss. Not a peck, but a long deep pleasurable kiss. I could lose myself in him just now, like the whole world revolves round us. Two lovers.

The doorbell rings, it must be the first guest. The surge of desire continues in me, and I can feel myself blushing. James's face is a beacon, his eyes bright with happiness, his cheeks flushed and his hair ruffled where I put my hand through it.

"I'd better get it. It's bound to be Derek, he's always early. I'll come back for you." He is out of the door before I can muster my brain into saying anything, but I follow in my wheelchair. I'm still slow and clumsy but I can get around given time, and I can't bear to let him out of my sight. Shaking with the need to be close to him, I make it to my door just as Derek is walking past. He sees my flushed face and looks back at James behind him, and he grins. Dear Derek, he is such a kind man. He would do anything for James, but he cannot understand a word I say. It's going to be tricky this evening. I am determined to make him understand, with or without someone to interpret for me, but it could just end up being a comedy of misunderstandings.

James catches hold of my wheelchair, as Derek says, "How are you Melissa? You look radiant." Never holds back does our Derek.

"Yehee yeh, yantyoo," I reply, mustering my best words to try and communicate with him.

He looks blank for a moment, and then, "Yes, I've tried that too, but it doesn't always work."

What on earth is he talking about? What did he think I said? Obviously not 'really well, thank you', but I hope it was nothing too embarrassing. He leads the way into James's snug sitting room, and we follow. James is wheeling me so I can't see his face. Perhaps he understands the exchange but he's not saying anything.

In spite of it having been a lovely morning, the weather turned cold and wet in the afternoon, so we decided to have our nibbles party inside. James made up a fire, and it is already burning with little bright flames – the smell of coal and wood filling his small Victorian parlour. Three occasional stacking tables are placed round the room laden with crisps, nuts, olives, and cheesy sticks. It's already quite warm in here, and I'm hoping this will explain why my cheeks are so red.

James sets me by the door so I can give the royal handshake and test people's comprehension as they enter.

"Red or white?" he asks Derek, and goes off into the kitchen to fetch our drinks, leaving us to have our misunderstandings.

I try a new tack. "Yot av ooh been doon day?" I am really impressed with myself – a six word phrase and clear at that.

"Yes, I saw that too. Don't usually watch the TV during the day, but couldn't miss that. Almost a dead heat, don't you agree? I just don't know how they work these things out at sea."

Oh dear, we really are at sea, and I'll never find out 'what he's been doing today'. I need my iPad, and it's in my room.

I turn my chair to go and get it, but James comes back with a tray of glasses and I nearly collide with him. "I bad," I mutter, explaining my need.

"No you're not, you're doing really well," Derek pipes up.

"Your iPad? I'll get it." James puts the tray down on an occasional table and pops into my room. So easy for him. I'm feeling exhausted and frustrated at the same time. Putting those earrings in took more out of me than I realised. If it wasn't for a certain sense of humour that I'm lucky enough to possess, I'd probably be crying all the time!

I like Derek. For all his inability to understand me, he is a caring soul. Thank god though, that he doesn't work in a caring profession. He's a designer. He designs cars, and I have become oddly, or perhaps not so oddly, interested in something that can move me from A to B in this dependent life of mine. Anything from large four-wheel drives to tiny eco cars like James's. Personally, I have become a Mr Toad in my dreams and rather fancy the sporty number that does 0-60 in five seconds. But what I really long for, if I'm being honest with myself, is that feel of being on a bicycle again - wind on my face, legs whirring round as I speed downhill. One moment, and it's gone.

Anyway, now I can talk cars with Derek until the others turn up. Even so, the iPad option is pretty slow. I have to concentrate hard to make my fingers go to the right keys, and I have this odd loss of spatial awareness which means I keep having to look for letters that I should know automatically.

I wheel myself over and start the conversation with my mechanical voice jerking out of the iPad's tiny speakers. A miniature miracle, but it's not me. I'm analogue, not digital.

After the opening gambit of "How is work? What are you d-e-s-i-g-n-i-n-g (difficult word – took me a while to find that one) now?" We can use pictures on the net to communicate by oohs and ahs, and are happily involved in a trawl through car-cabin

106

designs – Derek explaining what he is doing by showing me existing models. Space-age or retro? The Mr Toad in me prefers retro – a memory of old cars but with all the modern convenience of comfort and reliability. James's car is space age. Every fuel-saving gismo is packed into its small sleek body. But it has no soul, no roar, as it glides effortlessly around. Come to think of it, it's just as well I was hit by his previous eco car. If it had been a four-by-four it would probably have been curtains for me.

We are so wrapped up in our discussion that the first thing I notice are her legs. Wow, lovely legs. I look up and there is Cathy, dressed immaculately in pink. Pink jacket, pink skirt, pink shoes. I look up into her smiling face. She is young for sixty, but I still have to swallow a feeling of envy. She mothered James after his bereavement, and it has made them close. I want to mother James. I want to walk about on lovely legs in immaculate pink. I look down at my knees concealed under a sensible long skirt – anything short could be embarrassing as I'm not always sure what I'm doing with my legs.

"How are you?" she says, with a slightly West Country lilt.

"Dettin an oday." I reply automatically.

"Getting on OK?" she repeats back to me. I shouldn't feel irritated, she's really good at understanding me, but all the same it is so humiliating.

"Yes, det my eareens een on I oon."

"Got your earrings in yourself. That's great."

I mentally grind my teeth. Clever little girl. But be fair, what else could she say? "About bloody time too!" No, she's very clued up and knows something of the effort that my earring insertion would have caused.

She hands me my drink, raspberry and apple juice. No wine for me. My cerebellum can do without any more challenges thank you. And I haven't forgotten what a couple of halves of beer did for me.

Gradually the little sitting room fills up, and as there aren't enough chairs to go round, people stand up to talk, and all of a sudden I find myself excluded. Wheelchairs are like that. They bring you up to belly button height, but nobody talks or even listens through their belly button so that's that. The room is getting a bit hot too, so I feel I have an excuse for going out for some fresh air. I manage to get out of the door without running over anyone's toes, and I fumble my way out of the back door and into the garden.

It's a bit chilly out here. Despite being so-called summer, there's a cold wind spoiling any sense of a balmy warm evening. I look up. Clouds threaten - grey contrasting with the blue of this morning when everything looked so hopeful. I feel the sobs coming up from my depths, and it's no good. I can't stop it. I'm crying. Like a door slammed in my face, my past life is taken from me. And now…

"D-d-d-d-don't cry," says a voice behind me.

I turn and see a diminutive figure. Carl, I think his name is. He seemed very shy and scuttled off to the kitchen to help James as soon as he'd been introduced.

"Ahh-ah-are you alright?"

"No, sad." Two clear words for once. I look at him gratefully. A handsome little man, though his head looks too big for his body. A great shock of wavy hair sticks out at all angles, and he has a gold earring in his left earlobe. He picks up a battered old chair and comes to sit next to me. Two people with speech challenges. This should be some conversation. "Don't be so bitter," a voice says inside my head.

He looks at me sadly. There's not much to say. We're both excluded from the party, and now we're out in the cold wind and it's starting to drizzle.

Silence.

It's interesting how being with someone and just being silent can be so comforting. For both of us, making conversation – even just talking – is a huge effort. Now we can just sit in companionable silence, listening to the rain and watching our feet get wet, unprotected by the porch. The hubbub from the sitting room comes out to us, but we are better off out here. We are not understood in there; despite all best efforts we are barred from parties by our mouths.

Later, I will cuddle with James – I hope. Then, it comes to me that this is a very strange one-way relationship. He has taken me in, he is looking after me, he is making huge sacrifices. Why? Is it just simply love? Can I trust it? Or is he acting something out? His loss being made bearable by someone to look after. I am so much in his power. I never looked at it quite this way before: I have no independence, I rely on him entirely, and there is so much I don't know. This is very risky, and my fear is fuelled by his absence. He is in the middle of the party and he hasn't even noticed that I've gone. Oh, I can't bear this dependence.

With a sigh, my companion looks at his wet feet. "W-w-w-well, I-I-I-I'd better be g… g…" He gives up and gives me a hopeless look.

I smile at him, "Yant oo or sittin yi me," I say.

He looks puzzled for a moment and then, "Mmmm… mmm… mmmy pleasure," he says with a smile spreading across his handsome face. I pray someone will find him. He is a jewel, not mine, but definitely someone's. Somewhere. He doesn't attempt a goodbye, but just gives me a little wave and retreats into the house.

I sit and ponder my position for a while, wondering what to do – how I feel. Then turn my wheelchair and go back into the house. I look in through the door of the sitting room and see James in animated conversation with an attractive woman that I don't know. His face is flushed with wine and happiness. He is at home and he looks whole. Gone is his worried frown. He looks young and vigorous – the most attractive man I have ever seen, and I long to go over to him and tell him he's beautiful, but before I know it I'm propelling myself down the corridor to my room.

Isn't that what they say about horses? Their first instinct is flight, escape, which is what makes them always potentially dangerous, always ready to throw you off. Self-protection is their strongest urge, and when you ride them there is always this struggle going on inside them – to throw you off, or to bond with you.

I'm that horse. A strange thing to say when I'm in a wheelchair, but I can't decide whether to trust him or escape. That woman just now. Why was he so happy talking to her? Don't I do that for him? I move across the room to the mirror and see my face. Sad with tear stains. The muscles drawn down making me almost ugly. Those two earrings mocking me with their pathetic attempt at cheering up this sad sight.

The earrings. The ones he gave me earlier. Where are they now? Are they on the floor? Have I run over them – uncaring? I begin to look around my room, panic coming from nowhere. I must have them, I must touch them. Then maybe I will know. Out of the corner of my eye I catch a glimpse of something black. It's on the mantelpiece above the unused fireplace. The little black box he hid behind his back. I reach up and take it off the shelf, fumbling to open it without spilling its contents on the floor again. With trembling hands I manage to ease the lid off, and there they are – two diamonds twinkling up at me from their black velvet cushion. I look at them carefully, trying to find a clue as to who they were really meant for. Everything about the box looks new. It smells new, there is no sign of dust on it. With great care I manage to pick a stud up between my finger and thumb and place it on the palm of my left hand. The diamond is set in petals like a tiny flower, and as I look closer, I can see that each petal is made of an 'm'. Such a tiny detail, I thank God that I have such good eyesight. The one bit of me that works well.

I feel a hand on my shoulder and nearly drop the stud. I was so absorbed I didn't hear anyone come in.

"Are you OK? I saw you'd gone out for some fresh air, but then you didn't come back. I missed you." James turns me round in my wheelchair to look at him. He is glowing with happiness, his face radiant. "So you had to see them again. Do you like them?"

"I yuv yem. I yuv oo." I feel his warm hands on my face. And he crouches down and kisses me – long and warm, and in this moment my mood turns. I could lose myself in his hands. Right now, I need him completely, without question. Flushed now, I look up at him. He was happy because of me, because of us, and there was I wondering whether he wanted his freedom.

"Let's go back to the party. There's someone I want you to meet." He wheels me back to the sitting room, the hubbub dies down as we enter and all eyes are on us. The room is transformed, it is our room, these are our guests. I am not a little girl to be shoved in the corner somewhere. The overpowering crowd that I left has turned into a manageable group of ten people. And now I can meet them from a different place.

The guests that I hadn't met while I hid outside are introduced to me. And one in particular, the attractive woman that I saw James talking to is obviously the person I am meant to meet. She is very fit-looking, with a pretty face. Her features are small, jewel-like. Her eyes are dark brown, but piercing rather than soft. She has a ready smile, but also a firm look of someone who is used to helping people do things that are hard for them.

"This is Georgie. She's from Australia. You're going to her clinic on Monday."

Therapies and Memories

Chapter 14

Perth. I don't know how I came to be here, how it was paid for, but here I am. Driving south down a nearly empty dual carriageway. The first thing that strikes me is the light. It has an eagle-eye quality. So clear, like all the colours have been washed and ironed and they have come out bright and new. The air is different too, fresh, warm and toasty. There is a calmness about all this - so few cars, nobody breaking the speed limit. Long distances, why the rush? Time to just be, in my casement of plastic and metal as I cruise along getting closer to my destination.

After the gruelling flight on the grumpiest airline I have ever known, and before that, the terrible pain of losing my baby, this is so healing, so soft. I am going to a lake, and I'm going to stay in a cabin. And there's food there and people who will look after me. I pass signs advertising wineries. Margaret River. And I'm still going south. The trees get taller and I'm going through forest. The green light bouncing off my car windows. Fresh, cool.

I find the track which leads off to the lake, and on the way to my cabin I stop at a shack of a shop, and the first thing I hear:

"G'Day."

Wake up. Oh no, it's Monday. Time to go. Such a rush. James helps me into my clothes. Loose sweatshirt and joggers. We are going to physio. There is a lump in my throat. My heart is racing. Nightmare number one coming back. We arrive at the clinic. It's modern, cool, and fresh looking. We are welcomed by a woman in her fifties. Still fit, still slim. Long grey curly hair. Striking chiselled face. "You look fabulous," I want to say, but I can't speak for terror. No stand-up reception desk, just a tasteful dark oak table in the cool room. We wait, James sitting by me trying to interest me in the various right-wing trash that they have

115

displayed for waiting patients. Then I see it, a travel magazine. 'Explore Oz' on the cover. I reach out a shaking hand.

"Yat one bees."

And I'm back there.

The track up to my cabin is shaded by karri trees, there is a deep smell of lush warm vegetation coming through the open car window. I park on earth, and walk through the shady back porch to the rear of the cabin. There is firewood and an axe just by the doorway, and I open the insect screen and unlock my door. My door for two weeks. The cabin has a high roof, and through the screen at the front I see I have a long balcony looking down to the lake. As I walk onto it a group of bright green parakeets flutters up into the trees. I will sit out here a lot, but first, I'm hungry. Back inside the cabin there are vouchers for various meals, and I pick one up: 'Kangaroo steak with chips and beany salad.' Sounds interesting, but can I eat a kangaroo? I walk down to the lakeside restaurant – another shack, but long and low with a balcony right on the lake. I wait to be taken to my table.

"This way please."

Oh god, this is it. The first attempt at walking since my fall in the hospital. I have been putting it off, saying I'm not ready. But finally James has found someone who knows about my cerebellum, someone who specialises in my kind of injury. Georgie.

She looks harder-edged in her physio room wearing her t-shirt and tracksuit trousers. Her piercing eyes have a dark-steel look, and I feel she is not going to let me get away with excuses and tears. But first comes some pleasure. She massages my feet and legs with strong hands, knowing exactly how to switch on my muscles. The relief after all the aches I have

116

felt in my wheelchair-bound life is wonderful. I feel the blood flowing through the veins in my legs. The numbness and feeling of weakness is going away and I feel a resurgence of the old Melissa-legs. Those cycling legs that were once so fit.

"Now, let's see you stand." There are rails on both sides of me and I can use these to raise myself to standing. I have had a lot of practice using my arms to get on and off the loo, though I have avoided standing completely upright for any longer than I need to.

"It's really important for you to stand upright. It gives the cerebellum the right messages – fires it up. Human beings are meant to stand. Their brains and nervous system work that way, so standing and balancing are your way back to speech, coordination and all the things that aren't working for you at the moment." The way she says this, there is no doubt in her voice that all these things will work if I get myself back on my feet. So I grip the bars, take a deep breath and stand up.

"Stand up tall like a karri," I say to myself.

I climb the tallest karri tree in that part of Australia. There are metal pegs set in the trunk going round it like a spiral ladder, and I clamber up and round gripping the pegs tightly with my hands and stepping cautiously with my feet. I can see through the pegs down to the ground which is getting further and further away, and I'm beginning to wonder if I suffer from vertigo. I'm halfway up now and I'm stuck - clinging for dear life as the world goes round and round.

"Nobody has died climbing this karri tree," a voice says inside my head.

"There's always a first time," I reply, "and two people have had heart attacks afterwards."

"Oh come on, you're young and fit, get up to the top and see the view." I start to move again, stiffly this time, up and round,

round and up. Will I meet Mr Happy at the top? Perhaps I'll be Mrs Happy.

Finally I'm there at the top, and I take my time to look down. No, don't look down, look out into the Australian countryside. See the hills and trees and rivers and feel God at your elbow. Satan may have tried to tempt Jesus, but he's not tempting me – there's no way I'm going to jump.

"C'mon."

I am standing, gripping onto the bars, looking at the soft light coming through the windows at the other end of the room. I've done it, I'm up.

"That's great, now look around you, look at the poster on your right, yes the whale. Now look forward again at the window. Now look left at the elephant." Big creatures, she likes big creatures.

"Now sit down and have a rest."

With strong expert hands she supports me as I sit down into the security of my wheelchair. I did it. I felt a bit sick and dizzy, but by looking out instead of down I managed it.

"Let's try that again."

I stand up, sit down, stand up, sit down, over and over again. Deliberately, with a rest in between, but repetitively. I don't like this repetition. Something in my brain says this is wrong. I long to say "leave me alone," but something about Georgie's confidence makes me keep going. I know if I was a child I would play up and refuse. It's odd, it almost hurts, not physically, but like a painful twist in my nervous system. Ugh.

At last we stop, and I feel the unexpected urge to hit something. She wheels me over to face the wall.

"Push against the wall as hard as you can. This kind of work can be upsetting and make you feel angry." She stands behind me to stop my wheelchair from moving back.

As I push with all my strength my anger drains away, and I get the satisfying feeling of knowing where my head is after all those ups and downs.

I am sitting by the lake, there is a red glow still in the sky, and an open fire by the barbecue. Strangely, the whole barbecue thing in Oz is very modern. None of this cooking on the front grill of your series II Land Rover. Back in the seventies the Aussies were outraged when the series III came out with a plastic grill. 'What can you do with that, mate? Out in the bush, no barbie?' But now they have a public box that you barbecue on. All very neat and clean. A bit like an outdoors Aga. But no wood smoke – no carcinogens. So the open fire makes up for it, and we sit round the fire munching our x-burgers in the gathering gloom.

Someone has brought a guitar along, and they start to sing in a pleasant drawly kind of way. Then someone else gets out a ukulele, and a high strumming fills the night. Very south-seas feel. Where's the didgeridoo? I wonder. There is a rustle and a strange clang of metal just out of sight on the edge of the fire circle. I catch a glimpse of something square and steel – thin and solid. What on earth? A strange wang-a-wong starts up. Sound bubbles fill my head, and a compulsive rhythm takes over the night. Low and funny, it reminds me of Rolf Harris. That's it! But what's it called? The music grows, half humorous, half strange in the half-light. I feel the urge to get up and dance by the lake. Pagan, sensual, worshipping the god Pan. Others feel the same and we rise in a circle and dance a dance we never knew. We don't know how we do it, and will never know again. But now we are in it and the moon is glinting on the lake, the tall karri trees all around watch us in silent sentience. We dance for ages, weaving in and out in asymmetrical patterns. Heads high, heads low. Until as one we stop and sit down, exhausted.

"What was that?" I ask a shadowy neighbour as she hands me

a beer.

"The spirit of Oz I suppose."

"No, I mean that strange wobbly sound."

"Oh, a wobble board."

I knew it was too good to be true. The clock in the physio room shows that I am only halfway through the session. Back to the rails. What now? Georgie brings out a wooden circular board about two feet across, and places it on the floor just in front of me. It wobbles. Though it is flat on the upper surface, it is curved underneath so that if you stand on it you will wobble.

"A wobble board," says Georgie.

I stare down at it in disbelief. What kind of diabolical torture is this? Can she really expect me to step onto that thing when I can scarcely stand up at all? Her strong hands guide me up and onto its non-slip surface. And, terrified, I begin to wobble.

I have walked round the lake to the farthest point from my cabin. The sunbeams shaft through the tall trees. Their roots sometimes invading the path. I can hear a rushing, roaring sound ahead gradually invading the peace of the quiet forest. I know there is a waterfall on my walk, spectacular, according to the leaflet, but when I find myself looking up into the descending tower of water I am lost. There is no top to this tower. It goes up for ever, out of sight in the mist created by its own spray. Lost in wonder, I look and look. Absorbed in the roar and wetness. The ferocity of water pounding down. I feel at one with it. Lost in it.

Then I look ahead and see the gorge that this relentless water has made. Again it disappears into a mist. A rope bridge spans this bottomless void and I must cross it if I am to continue my journey round the lake. Set against the massive forces of nature that surround it, the bridge looks frail and spindly – just a little bit of knotted rope. Cautiously, I walk towards the bridge, fearing that the ground will give way at any moment and that I will plunge to my death in the misty gloom below. There are rope rails on either side just above waist height and I grasp these and take a step onto the bridge. It sways slightly under my weight. I don't want to let go of the rope rails, and I am frozen for a moment, unable to move any further. I wish there was someone else here to go first and show me that it can be done.

Then, in my head, reason takes over. "Lots of people have crossed this bridge before you. It must be perfectly safe."

But then another voice points out, "There's always a first time. It might be you that has the fatal accident."

In the end reason persuades me to go onto the bridge. There is also the fear of looking a fool being stuck on the edge. My hands ache from gripping the rough rope, and they chafe as I slide them along and take my first step. The bridge sways slightly again, and I wonder what it will be like when I reach the middle. Worse, certainly. I take another step, then another. With each step I sway a bit more, and then I look down. The floor of the bridge is made from wooden slats, and although my feet won't go through the gaps between them, I can see the depths below. A steam of spray parts to show me jagged rocks and a faint glint of water far, far below.

I shouldn't have done that. My head starts to spin and I feel like I'm going to faint. I'm getting near the middle of the bridge now, and it's swaying more and more as I move. Terror really takes over as I swing from side to side suspended over the gorge. Then I feel the bridge sway differently, no longer with the rhythm of my movement. Someone else is on it.

"You OK?" A warm male Australian voice is behind me. "Been over this loads of times. Perfectly safe."

I shake my head in response. Fear has momentarily caused a loss of speech.

"Look, just move one hand then step and then move the other..."

"But we're both on the bridge," I stammer, finding my voice. "Won't it collapse with our weight?"

"I've taken groups of kids over here. Ten at once. It's strong enough to support an army."

I move a hand forwards. Part of me is convinced by this Aussie lunatic.

"Now look ahead, not down."

Slowly, painfully, I make my way to the other side. My rescuer keeps just behind me, encouraging me all the way across. I get my feet onto solid ground and turn to thank him. There's no-one there, just the gently swaying bridge.

"Now, try and see if you can balance." Georgie is by me and I feel her support through my clenched up hands and arms. The vortex is below me.

"Look ahead of you."

I feel the wobbling get less, and calm down a little.

"Now, put your weight into your right leg."

Shakily, I do this. I wobble down to the right and then stop. OK so far.

"Now put your weight into your left leg."

The hokey-cokey! Okey-dokey. I manage this and sink shakily down to the left side. We do this again and I feel more confident. But then the third time I suddenly feel my weight going backwards. I'm going to fall.

I scream. She's there. She's holding me. My terror subsides but I feel weak.

"I think that's enough. You've done really well." She guides me off the wobble board and into my wheelchair which was only just behind me.

"More heavy work, and then a massage to finish."

So I push against the wall and feel relief as the pent up anger and fear ebbs away. Then, oh joy, the massage. I sink into babyhood and let her wring out the tension from my arms, shoulders and legs.

Chapter 15

Turn back young Leonard do not venture in,
For there's deep and false water in the Lake of Marsh Green.

Now it's always struck me as interesting that I can sometimes be so freaked by heights, but am always quite happy to be in water with unknown depths beneath me. Lakes are dangerous places to bathe. They can often be much colder and deeper than you expect, and people drown simply because their bodies cramp up with the cold and they sink like a stone.

I am up early this morning. The Australian sun is just peaking over the treetops by the lake, and I'm going to be a bit naughty. I have got hold of a wetsuit, and I am going to swim out into the lake away from the roped off safety area. With the wetsuit on I am hoping that I will be sufficiently protected against the cold, and so will not cramp up. I also have a buoyancy aid with me, just in case. The water feels cold to my feet as I walk in, and I shiver, even in the warmth of my wetsuit, wondering whether I should just give up on this idea. But the morning is perfect, no-one around, and I know I'll just want to do it tomorrow if I don't do it now.

I slide into the water, and my expert swimming reflexes take over. That beauty of gliding through water – the pulse, the breathing, all physical systems combined in one movement. Before I've even thought about it, I'm at the diving platform at the edge of the safe swimming area. I pull myself up onto it, feeling the full weight of earth's gravity for a moment, and then dive off the other side and into the unknown.

The weeks have gone by and I am slowly responding to the repetitive physio sessions. Georgie pushes me to my limits, but even though I am making good progress, there is a huge obstacle for me to overcome. My fear of falling. Any unexpected wobble will bring on my panic. It's like a phobia, but we know that part of it is my brain telling me that I am going to fall into a chasm. Not just onto the floor or into Georgie's arms, but a thousand feet to my death. This is the message, and it's very difficult to override it. As soon as this happens, it will take us a long time in the session to get my confidence back again.

But now we are going to try something new: aqua-therapy. James and Georgie both knew that I loved swimming, but the problem was how to get me into a pool without me completely freaking out on the way. In the end, Georgie decided that we'd just try it, and see if I would calm down sufficiently to gain from the effects of the weight-bearing water.

They have helped me into a tight wetsuit to give my muscles and nerves more feedback. Also it will give me support in case of an ataxic moment – the involuntary floppiness that can happen especially if I'm tired. My arms and legs are exposed but my core is encased in neoprene.

We get to the poolside using my wheelchair, but now I have to get up - Georgie supporting me on one side, and Jane the aqua-therapist on the other.

"I think the steps will be too much for you." Jane is from Yorkshire. She's in her forties and looks like she's swum all her life. Her arms and shoulders look strong and reassuring, and she has that solid physicality that comes with being a mother and carrying children, shopping, in fact everything. I am sure she will be able to carry me in the water.

Gently the two of them lower me down onto the floor by the side of the pool. They help me slide on my bum so that my legs can drop down into the water. It feels warm and inviting, and I sit there with the two of them on either side of me, looking down at the gentle ripples on the surface of the pool. A certain longing takes hold of me and all I want to do is to slide in and swim away, but I have no idea whether my damaged reflexes will let

126

me do it. Instead, Jane gets into the water and Georgie gently helps me down into her arms.

I lie on my back, afloat over a mass of water, unknown depths beneath me. I can see a fringe of karri trees all around me. It encloses me, gently lulling me into a sense of security. I turn and swim out towards the middle of the lake, and as I do so I feel the increasing cold. Something inside me is telling me to turn back, but I have come this far and I want to be there – right in the middle, surrounded by masses of water. A shadow crosses overhead, I am frightened for a moment, but as I look up, it is only an old kookaburra flapping out looking for God-knows-what.

I am definitely getting colder now...

Wow, this is something else. The water supports me, I feel... safe...er. But! Moving legs through all this heavy water is hard... hard. I think I have moved. Feedback through muscles tells me that definitely something has happened. Georgie (bless her) on one side, and the yet-to-be-discovered and trusted Jane on the other. Yes, I actually moved through this treacle-like substance. So much safer than that hard floor I can hit at any moment. I lurch forward giving them no warning, and... I go under!

It's too cold. I can feel my muscles beginning to seize up. I have forgotten my buoyancy aid, left it on the diving platform. I turn and try to swim for the bank. Any bank where the water is shallower and warmer will do. But a strong current is pulling me into the middle. I struggle with it but the cramp in my legs makes it impossible. My arms are still working; though it is not enough to work against the current, they are keeping me afloat. I feel the bitter cold seeping through my thin wetsuit and I know I am going to die. The current pulls me inexorably into the deepest coldest part of the lake and I'm going down. I take a deep breath, the

127

cramp and force of water take me under, I am sinking, sinking...

Strong hands lift me spluttering, "You're not ready to go it alone." A strong Yorkshire accent in my ear, then, "How'd she do that?" to Georgie on my other side. Jane has forgotten that I'm human, and is doing that talking-as-though-I-weren't-there thing.

"Use do sweem ayot," I gasp, determined to be part of this exchange.

"What did she say?"

"Was a good swimmer."

I'm still not present to them. Just an object to be manoeuvred. Rage takes me and I shout, "Teck te meee!" And I struggle with them with such force that they nearly lose me again.

"We'd better get her out, she's panicking," Jane shouts.

I don't want to get out, I just want to be treated like a human being. My arms are strong from all the wheelchair work, and they find it harder to move me than they expected. We all end up at the side of the pool panting with the exertion.

"What the fuck is going on?" Jane is losing it. Her grip on my arm is painfully tight and I can feel a mixture of panic and anger surging through. She is an experienced aqua-therapist but she's never had to deal with someone like me. Georgie, on the other hand, is calmer.

"She... er... you hate being talked over, as though you're not there. You said 'talk to me', is that right?"

I nod, not trusting my crap vowels. I begin to calm down, I am human again. There are three of us.

"So that's it. Listen sunshine, we have to talk about you as we are doing this. You will just have to be patient." Jane's grip has lessened slightly, but she is still hurting me. I look at Georgie, and I see a look of resignation on her face. We need a different aqua-therapist. 'Sunshine' indeed. End of relationship.

"I think we had better stop for now," Georgie says. I agree – I want to be in the water. I know that it is the way forward, but not with this person.

I'm on the shore of the lake, gasping for breath. How did I get there? Last thing I knew I was drowning, and now I'm dragging my body painfully out of the water and into the rooty undergrowth that surrounds this part of the lake. The current must have carried me rapidly past the middle of the lake and to the edge. First the rope bridge experience and then this. This place is weird.

Painful feeling is coming back into my legs, and I rub them weakly to try and get the circulation going. For the moment I am a stranded whale, but the sun is beginning to come up over the trees and it will warm me back into life.

"What the fuck?" A woman's voice with a strong Australian accent just behind me. She's struggling through the undergrowth towards me.

"You OK?"

I nod, shivering too much to say anything.

"She's over here! She's alive!"

I'm alive and I'm in trouble. Soon I am wrapped up in blankets and carried back to the resort, where the on-site nurse checks me over while they wait for a doctor to arrive. I have survived hypothermia and will soon be up and running, but the resort people are not amused.

"We thought you had committed suicide," the resort manager puts it bluntly. "Pull another trick like that and we will send you home."

I am a naughty child. I have caused a lot of people a lot of trouble. I blink back tears of shame and anger. I will make it up to them somehow.

In his arms. I'm back in his arms. Safe again, please come with

129

me to find a decent aqua-therapist. I need you.

Georgie has had quite a conversation with James. She's angry, and a bit ashamed as she found the dreaded Jane in the first place. But I trust her and forgive her. The whole therapies thing is a minefield – what's good for one person is no good for another. Still, I bet Georgie had never heard her say 'sunshine' like that. Yuck, I feel sick at the thought.

We lie side by side looking up at the ceiling, and suddenly I feel claustrophobic. I want to get out of my room, out of this house, out of my wheelchair, and into freedom. This sudden urge makes me cry – I bury my face in James's chest and sob. He holds me and, with that part of my mind that isn't crying, I wonder what he's thinking. Abruptly I push away from him and look him straight in the face.

"I wanna fly." Then the sobs take over and I can't say anything for some time.

Chapter 16

Aqua-therapy, physiotherapy, occupational therapy, speech therapy, therapy-therapy. Time goes by and I improve – not steadily like a train going up Snowdon, but in fits and starts – sometimes actually going backwards, and then leaping forwards unexpectedly. They say the only thing we can expect about my recovery is that it will do the unexpected. The damaged links from my nervous system and main brain to my cerebellum are faulty, but they are gradually finding alternative routes and channels, and one of the most confusing things is that suddenly, overnight a new neuro-pathway will be constructed and I can do something that I never thought I would be able to do again. This is made even more confusing by the relearning I have done in some areas that is now rendered obsolete. Take speech for instance. Having struggled with the simplest of phrases, I unexpectedly come out with sentences perfectly formed as if from nowhere. My newly learnt way of speaking – incomprehensible to many well-meaning friends – still kicks in, but now I realise that if I just let it happen, my old speech patterns will work and the world of conversation will open up to me again. But it hurts. It's like a peculiar twist in my guts. It makes me shiver, feel slightly sick, and very angry all at the same time. All that relearning and now my brain's doing it for me. Perfectly.

I should be praising God, singing alleluias, and jumping for pure joy. I really am grateful, honestly. I know of others with my kind of damage who never recover, and so many other brain injuries that render you totally incapable, sometimes unreachable. I am one of the lucky ones. And I'm loved. But wherever you are, isn't it funny how there's always problems, bitterness, fears to overcome. I guess that's our pathway, our destiny. There's no escape from our selves. We have to live through whatever we throw at ourselves, whatever patterns we have refused to tackle in our lives. Ignore yourself at your peril.

One part of my 'damage' that refuses to change is my fear of falling. The sickness, the feeling of an endless fall into a bottomless pit is always with me if I wobble or lose my balance. Georgie says my core strength is there now, and that I can support myself well. But I still have the odd bout of ataxia. This evil and debilitating thing – this sudden weakness in my muscles that can happen at any time, but particularly when I'm tired. Ataxia means that I can never quite trust my body to stay upright all the time, and so, put together with my extreme fear of falling, it thoroughly hampers my progress out of the wheelchair and into independent walking. I think that the ataxia and the fear of falling all come in the same neurological package, so I shouldn't blame myself too much. I still cry every time it happens.

I can remember a girl who lived on the edge like this. Survival was her edge. Getting enough to eat, trying to make a relationship work. Trying to hold down a job. Trying to have a baby.

After the fire they all went into a cold hell. Each one trapped in their own too private grief, hugging the pain and guilt to themselves like holding burning hot brands to their chests, or running into the salt sea with their open wounds. Their suffering was obsessive and had nowhere to go except round and round.

How did the fire start? Was it a duvet falling on an old electric fire? Was it uncle Don's smoking habit? Or did the boys make a camp fire in the attic? They never really knew.

Her father was the first one to break out of their circle of ashes. No longer able to cope with the dull office drudgery of the civil service, he got a job as a lorry driver, preferring the slow grind of manoeuvring large lorries round our small British roads. Sometimes he escaped to the Continent on a long haul and would be away for days. His bleak mind dwelt on the minute measurements needed to get a large object through small spaces. He took pride in his accuracy, and his thoughts were taken up with millimetres and wing mirrors.

He would come home to a silent household. His wife a shadow hiding in the kitchen or in front of the television. Scuttling to and fro trying to keep them alive with her dull cooking. His daughter was growing up, and he began to notice her increasing beauty – she had that long-haired lithe-limbed look so reminiscent of the hippie girls of the late sixties. She was his only way in. The only chink of light in his dark cold home. They began to take walks together – they would never talk about the fire, or about the feelings that were buried in their concrete gardens.

School had become an anathema to her. She showed talent at sculpture, and buried herself in novels, but failed miserably in her exams.

So father and daughter walked and talked about books, and about the trees in the park. The powerful shapes and stories that surrounded them on all sides. So much to look at, so much potential for a young creative mind. The more time he spent with her, the more he came to love her not just as his daughter but as another person.

The problem was that he became too close, too needed, too needy. He was relying on her like a spouse. She relied on him as a lover. But there was no real tangible sexual love between them, father and daughter as they were. It was all concealed in the odd hug that was seconds too long, or the odd inappropriate kiss on the lips. But love each other they did, more than they should, and eventually her father gathered all his strength and courage and left. Moved out. Drove his lorry off into the night.

She left her home too. A home that was horribly scarred by a fire. Couldn't bear it any more. Found the first man that was free and hooked up with him. Her father gone now she would do anything to get away from that cold hell of grief.

His name was David and he was good enough. He worked on farms and they lived together in tied cottages, working a season then moving on. The cottages looked pretty from the outside, but they were often dank, mouldy and rat-ridden on the inside.

They held hands, they made love, they went to the pub, he drank too much. Not that this made him violent, it just slowed him down in the morning. Slowed him down in life.

Not much money left to pay for food. She tried making little sculptures to sell, but to no avail, so she went out and found whatever work there was – shop assistant, waitress, some farm work. All paid below the minimum wage. But they ate. Tesco two-for-one. End-of-market sell-offs. Fruit in season, cheap veg, cheap meat, bread and milk, and if they were lucky real eggs from the locals. They shared their food, unintentionally, with the rats and mice. It was amazing how clever and discreet the rats could be. Things would disappear without a trace. No droppings, no mess. The rats, contrary to popular belief, were fastidious private creatures. You wouldn't know they were there if they didn't steal your food. Mice on the other hand were messy, left droppings everywhere, and could often be interrupted during their midnight raids, scuttling across the floor to hide in a corner, only to come out again a minute later forgetting the very recent threat.

Winters were the worst. The farm cottages had no insulation, no double glazing. Only primitive electric heating and small open fires. Keeping warm and dry was a constant problem. Scavenging fallen branches would be one way, if there was a wood close by. Going to the pub was very attractive then. Any pub would do. She would nurse her two half pints while David drank away their food and fuel. They were warm till chucking-out time, but then there was the walk home to the cold cottage.

One night she thought they would die. It was bitterly cold and it had snowed two days earlier. Now there was a crust of hard ice on top of the thick powdery snow. David was drunker than usual, and she was having a hard time keeping him upright. An unexpected drift caught them out and they both fell into a snow-filled hole. David was face down and seemed unconscious. He was too heavy for her to lift, she was up to her waist and was struggling to get out herself. They were like that for half an hour - him inert, her trying to pull him out. In the end he came to, and managed to muster enough strength to pull himself out of the ditch. They got home to their freezing house so cold and exhausted that all they could do was to lie down and cover themselves with the filthy rugs off the floor.

She left him then, and ended up on the streets in Oxford, begging in St Giles. A kind Blackfriar would drop a pound coin into her hat every now and then, and give her a smile. She came to know him and others like him who would also drop in the odd bit of generosity. So she would eventually have enough to eat, and stay at one of the hostels provided in that city of 'dreaming spires'. She kept away from drugs and prostitution - she was often approached, even threatened.

Then she met Daniel.

She was in the public library reading Hesse. She loved Hesse. So simple, so fluent to read, and yet such fine quality. She read *Siddhartha* four times. In a way she identified with the young prince who left all to go on his spiritual journey. Suffering, nearly starving, begging.

But this cold winter's afternoon she was tackling Hesse's most challenging work, *The Glass Bead Game*. She was enthralled by his description of a world so different. So intuitive, so far from the newspaper-driven society in which she just about managed to survive: she read of books, libraries, comfort, safety.

It was warm in the library after the cold Oxford streets, and she went to sleep, curled up in her plastic-covered chair.

Deep in a pool of wine I wait
For word's internment, for whose sake?
Neon light and plastic chair
The smell of books on heated air.

She shifts she stirs, this girl in rags
I see her beauty frail and fair.
Look at myself in clothes so neat
Look at this princess at my feet.

Her nails I notice are kept clean
Beneath her grubby clothes unseen
Her milk white skin shines out of sight
I would have her for just one night.

I curse the wine, the rancid thought
Of this sweet girl by my hands caught.
Free us all Lord from our chains
And let our souls fly, fly, fly.

Daniel wrote, and watched her sleep. He realised the pretension of his Renaissance style, could almost have sung it to his lute. He deleted the third verse, then the fourth, leaving the first two. Then he closed the file without saving it.

What was he doing? Music don, organist, single man, one bottle of wine down at two thirty in the afternoon looking at a street girl in the public library? Was he lost? He'd stumbled in there on the pretence of looking for a book about Buxtehude that he couldn't find in the university libraries. But really, why was he here writing poems on his laptop?

As he looked up, a door opened in the opposite wall, and a nondescript balding individual walked over to where Melissa was sleeping.

136

"I'll have to ask you to leave," he whispered to her with a harsh edge to his voice, looking round in an embarrassed way as though the entire population of the library had their eyes glued on him.

But getting no reaction from her, he said to Daniel urbanely. "We get them all the time – street people sleeping here, taking up the chairs, being a nuisance to library users." He paused for a moment. "Has she asked you for money?"

"No, no," Daniel was taken aback. "No, she's been reading Hesse – see," he pointed at the book on her lap. "She must have fallen asleep."

The man moved to shake her by the shoulder.

"No don't do that. The poor thing needs her sleep."

"Probably on drugs or drink; well she's not sleeping it off in here." The man was officious. He looked like a frog, blown up with its own pomposity.

"Listen, I've never seen someone on drugs reading Hesse's *The Glass Bead Game* before. Have you?" Daniel had stood up and was moving over to protect her. The bald man looked alarmed. Picking on shabby-looking street urchins was one thing, but this man looked respectable, for all the smell of wine on his breath.

"What's *The Glass Bead Game*? Some cult book I expect. These drug abusers are always finding some cranky book to fix their ideas on."

"Look, can't she just sleep while I keep an eye on her? I've got work to do," Daniel gestured at his laptop, "and I can make sure she does no harm when she wakes up."

"Library policy. No sleeping vagrants. Apart from anything else, they smell."

Daniel reflected that the only smell he could detect was that of plastic, and some kind of cheap air freshener.

The girl opened her eyes, looking round blurrily for a moment, and then abruptly sat bolt upright, her left hand searching for her bag. *The Glass Bead Game* fell onto the floor.

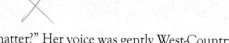

"Wha... what's the matter?" Her voice was gently West-Country. "Is... is it alright for me to read books here?"

"You'll have to leave." The official was immoveable. "We can't let you sleep here."

"But I only dozed off for a minute. I've been coming here regularly. I love this library – love reading. Adam said it was OK."

"Well it's Adam's day off." He was obviously even more irritated by the fact that his subordinate had been giving the likes of her permission to read books in his library. "You're going to have to go. Now come on, get up."

At this point Daniel intervened. Was it the wine that lent strength to his resolve? Or was there an angel about? He'd never know. He stepped into something entirely new when he took the man's arm.

"Now look here," his voice was vibrant with emotion. "I don't know what kind of librarian hasn't heard of *The Glass Bead Game*, but I will make a formal complaint to the... to the manager."

"I am the manager." His pompous face was red with anger. Everyone was looking at them. A typical English scene. No-one would make a move – too embarrassing –but they looked.

Daniel stepped back from the manager, and leaned forward towards the street girl. "Shall we go? I'll take you to somewhere else if you like."

She paused, looked at him, reluctant to trust him. Looking down, she picked up her tattered bag and stood up, ready to leave.

"Just a minute miss." Someone had called security, and here he was in person, in his uniform. "Can I just check your bag?"

"Oh for heaven's sake." Daniel was going to intervene again, but she handed the man her bag. They'd been through this before. The security man felt the bag for books and quickly handed it back to her.

"Shall I show you out miss?" They walked together out of the library door and down the stairs to the street with Daniel trailing behind. A fresh blast of wintery air met their faces as the security man opened the door.

The glass doors closed behind them – Melissa shuddered with the cold.

"Let me get you a coffee." Daniel said, "It's freezing out here."

"Can we go to a place that does herbal tea?"

Chapter 17

Standing in the car park outside M&S – I'm stuck. James has gone to the loo, and I thought I could manage to wheel myself to the car and get in without his help. Somehow I got it wrong – part of my problem is that I am really bad at judging distances. Sometimes I'm not even sure where my arms and legs end. Proprioception – we're working on it, Georgie and I, but at this moment it has let me down badly. So I thought I'd manoeuvred the wheelchair correctly so that I could just reach out and open the door to let myself in, but I'd got it wrong. I was too far away from the car, and worse than that, I'd not put the wheelchair brake on and it rolled away when I stood up leaving me with nothing to hold on to.

Stranded, with the fears beginning to take over, I feel like I'm on the point of a pin, high above the tarmac of the car park. I'm going to fall. I feel the nausea coming on. Last time this happened... I feel a hand take me by the elbow.

"Melissa. What happened to you?"

I look round to see Daniel.

He had a kind face. Slightly too much skin and jowl, but natural smile creases. Twinkly eyes, and nice bushy eyebrows beneath his receding hairline. Forties, she thought. University?

They sat in an old café. The windows had steamed up so they looked out at vague blobs moving by. People out in the cold.

"I'm Daniel," he held out his hand awkwardly across the table.

"Melissa." She took it firmly and felt his gentle grip. A gentle man?

"Melissa, well..." He didn't know what to say. How did you end up like this? He could hardly ask that – it sounded so brutal, so offensive. She'd had enough thrown at her in the last half-hour. Where to start? He'd always thought it polite to ask other people

141

about themselves as an opening to conversation. But this time...

"I'm a don. Music. I play the organ... er... and the lute. I am very interested in English Renaissance music..." he stumbled to a halt. He had been living in a sort of fantasy world so prevalent in this 'city of dreaming spires'. Now, across the table, was reality.

Melissa looked down at the Formica table top, unable to meet his eyes. Then she said something so quietly he couldn't hear it.

"Sorry?"

"Do you play any Dowland? Oh thank you," she whispered as the waitress put the pot of peppermint tea in front of her. "I love *In Darkness Let Me Dwell*. Have you played it?"

Daniel was taken aback.

"Yer... yes. I did it with Michael Chance years ago in the chapel. Loads of wood – perfect acoustic." *What is this girl? Why is she here like this?*

"Way to keep warm," as if in answer to his question. "Listen to music in the record shops. They seem to like Dowland in Blackwell's, but Michael Chance – wow."

There was a long silence while they sipped at their drinks. Daniel noticed how she poured her mint tea out so delicately. Drinking it too, with care – sniffing the aroma, holding the cup with both hands reverently like a grail. He sipped his double shot latte hardly tasting it. It was good, but he was so used to the good life, that it had almost lost all its flavour. Better have another one, he thought, sober up from the bottle of St Emelion that went down with lunch without him even noticing.

"Would you like another?" he asked beckoning over the waitress.

"No thanks," she indicated her pot, still half full.

"Another latte please, a double shot."

The waitress looked at Melissa, taking in her rags and sniffed slightly.

"Would you like something to eat?" Daniel realised that he hadn't offered her anything, and she was probably starving.

142

The waitress shifted from one leg to the other as though keen to get away from this polluting presence in her café.

"Do you do soup with bread?" Melissa looked directly at her.

"Mulligatawny. White or brown?"

"Brown please."

The waitress left, muttering something about soup kitchens. Daniel reflected that she could have been on the streets herself – the dividing line between poor and absolute poverty was so small. Mind you, if I continue consuming this amount of alcohol I'll probably end up on the streets myself. He thought of an afternoon seminar when he couldn't pronounce the word 'musician', it came out 'moozish...shun.' The thin edge of the wedge.

"You saved me, you know."

We are sitting in the café at M&S and I have been telling Daniel about my accident. James, who arrived too late to rescue me, recognised an old friendship, and discreetly slipped off to do some more shopping leaving us to catch up.

"No really." Daniel says. He looks much older – grey with his creased face filled with lines. He has a slight stoop now, but something in his face shows a kind of happiness and contentment that come from a fulfilled life.

"You saved *me*." I say. "Just now I thought, oh I thought I was going to fall. It's horrible that feeling. And then, all those years ago, when you found me in the library."

Daniel watched her dip her bread in her soup, and as he watched, a thought came into his mind. She could come and live with him – as a lodger. He didn't want anything else from her, did he? No. That would be it. He had room to spare. She could stay there and find her feet. He'd buy her some new clothes – provide her with food, give her a roof over her head. But how to persuade her that there were no strings attached.

143

"Would you like somewhere to live?"

She looked up at him startled, and started to get up from the table.

"No, don't go. I've got a spare room in my house that I rent to students," he told the lie on the spur of the moment. No good, she was out of the door in a flash leaving her bag of possessions behind her. He hastily put down his coffee, spilling some of it, picked up her bag and ran to the door. Looking out he saw her disappearing round the corner. They were in the covered market, alleyways everywhere. He ran to catch her up, hearing the outraged shout from the waitress behind him. Rounding the next corner, he nearly bumped into a burly man carrying a bread tray, but Melissa had vanished.

"I could have told you she'd do that!" The waitress was acidic on his return. "You can't trust them."

She, Melissa, doesn't trust me, he thought as he put down the money on the table.

It took him most of the afternoon to find her, half-concealed in a doorway outside Blackfriars. He held out her bag, and she grabbed it looking as though she was going to run again. Then she looked him full in the face, holding his gaze for a moment, searching for something in his eyes. She saw sadness, loss, and a gentleness. There was something missing, no relationship, an emptiness in his life.

"Where do you work?" Again she spoke almost in a whisper, as though she hardly used her voice.

"Just round the corner at St... Do you want to see?" The sadness in his face was replaced by a look of hope. She looked at him and nodded, and they went together, nudging their way through the crowds waiting for the lights on the corner. He led the way down the street and through the hallowed portals of the college.

"Afternoon Mr Brownlow." The porter in his lodge raised his eyebrows at the sight of Daniel's companion but made no comment.

Daniel led the way into the chapel. The smell of old stone and wood always gave him a feeling of home. Here, he could take charge. Hone a bunch of ragged students into a first-class choir. Play Bach on the beloved organ with its tracker action and flutey European-sounding pipes. Put on performances for whoever would care to come. He didn't mind – he knew that what he gave was good as long as he didn't drink too much.

"So..." Melissa whispered again, but the rich acoustic of the chapel picked up her sound and whisked it into corners and crevices. "This is where you work." She spun around, looking up at the ceiling with its ornately carved beams. A high fluted forest of fine work. She walked slowly up the nave looking from side to side, taking in the ornate carved woodwork. The pews with their crests, the memorial plaques on the walls, the fine panelling.

"Elizabethan?" She scarcely breathed the word.

"No, later – baroque. But look at this."

The west window was ablaze with light. Blues, rich reds and purples invaded the chapel with a glorious pandemonium of colour. She couldn't clearly see the subject of the stained-glass window, but she could tell it was comparatively recent. Piper? Chagall? It took her back to her studies in art at school, and suddenly she felt refreshed from her head down to her toes. What a medium, to tell a story and broadcast it with nature's light all over the walls of the grateful building.

She looked round in a reverie, her movement made the colours dance, and when she closed her eyes she could still see them even more clearly refracted from her retina.

The vibrations of the lowest pipes of the organ reached her then. Sonorous, deep, melodious but with a melancholy that she appreciated. The line repeated, but with another part, then another. Building to a fullness of tears. Sadness and glory mixed in a perpetual round of melody. The repeated pattern of the passacaglia pulled her into a world of true deep joyful sadness. She was in love, but it was with the music. She luxuriated in this bed of sound, the glory of the building resonating with colour and shape. All was brought together in this moment - sound, sight, smell, feeling. She spun round to catch the notes as they seemed to bounce off the walls and ceiling. She wanted it never to stop, but it did. There must be something else to follow, it felt incomplete.

Silence. She stood, still. The music still reflected in her mind like the light before it.

"Bach's C minor Passacaglia. Can't play the fugue, at least not after a bottle of wine." He sounded jaunty, but she detected something else behind it - he was moved, he clearly hadn't expected to come out with such a performance. She looked at him; he had tears in his eyes.

"Why the wine? You have so much... music. If it stops you playing it can't be good."

The first real sentence he'd got out of her and she was telling him.

"You got me off it, you know," he says.

I knew. A magical relationship between a celibate heavy drinker and a girl searching for family, for love. Not sex. Love. I loved him then, and I find that I still do now.

"But I was lost. I had no-one." My words come out – unbidden.

"Not just you."

"I know."

M&S was difficult for both of them - he had no idea what to buy for her. She wondered why she was committing herself by letting him buy her clothes. He wanted to leave her to it, and then pick up the bill at the end, but she insisted he follow her around approving this and that.

146

Jeans, t-shirts, jumpers were all OK, but when it came to pants, tights and bras, he left her to it, and pretended to study the men's clothes on the other side of the aisle. It was all very unsettling, she was so very attractive, that it almost physically hurt him.

A warm coat and sturdy shoes and they were done.

"I still love M&S you know."

"Haven't been to the one in Oxford for years." He sighs and I remember back to that time, seeing that poor man patiently following me round like a father. But he wasn't my father, and I loved him after a while.

They walked down St Aldates, over Folly Bridge and into the relative quietness of South Oxford. Victorian terraces, and a feeling of gentleness with just a few small shops. She wore her new coat over her rags. It had started to snow and she was glad of the extra warmth. What was she getting into? she wondered. She hoped Daniel was what he seemed – simply lonely and well-meaning. The urge to fly was still with her, and she would do so at the slightest sense of danger.

They passed a park and took a side road. Red-brick Victorian terraces lined both sides of the road.

"Here we are." Daniel fumbled in his pocket for his keys and unlocked the front door letting them into a narrow hallway.

Not much space, she reflected.

They put down their bags and he showed her into the living room. It was bigger that she expected, having been knocked through to the dining room at the rear. A comfortable sofa and chair in an old-fashioned flowery style clashed with horrible orangey-brown curtains that must have been there since the seventies. The room had a bare unloved feeling with its single light hanging from the ceiling, and the curtains were drawn giving it a gloom that added to the depression. She felt the urge to bolt then. The room made her feel trapped – she had spent so much time outside with space around her, and she suddenly felt intensely claustrophobic.

Instead of running she marched firmly up to the front windows and threw back the curtains. Light shafted in from the street lamps outside and she could see snow falling gently caught in the glow.

"I always keep them shut. Don't know why. Privacy I suppose." He sounded defensive, even hurt. He turned the light on in the kitchen which led straight back from the living room in a typical Victorian terrace layout. Dirty washing-up was piled up by the stainless steel sink. The cupboards were white chipboard with melamine tops, and a pile of empty bottles spilt over from a bin in the corner. The smell of stale coffee pervaded the room, and Melissa suppressed the urge to retch, reminded as she was of childhood car journeys when the only receptacle on offer to be sick in was a large used coffee mug.

"Would you like to see your room? I have been using it as a dumping ground for books. I really have been meaning to put up some shelves. Just haven't got round to it." His voice lost confidence as he spoke, becoming an apologetic mutter as he led the way up the narrow steep stairway to the first floor landing. Straight ahead she saw a bathroom, and turning along the landing there was a half-open door.

"This is it." He fumbled for the light switch and cursed softly as nothing happened.

She looked in. The floor was covered with books and music, all lit up by the evening urban glow coming in from outside. He stood aside for her as she stepped carefully over the books and looked out of the window. So this is it, she thought, my first room away from... home. There were no curtains and she looked out at a small garden backing onto a park. The sudden feeling of space surprised her, and she thought: I could live here.

Daniel had scrabbled around behind her and found a lamp by the single unmade bed. He switched it on.

148

"There. What do you think? Needs a bit of sorting."

"It's... lovely." She couldn't say more, a sudden feeling of homesickness combined with an odd gratitude made it impossible. She would have cried, and she didn't want to show him her emotion.

He was already bustling about picking up books and taking them out into the corridor. She helped him willingly, needing the comfort of doing something to get her through this pang, this palpable feeling of home. Together they stacked the books outside her room, leaving just enough space for him to get past to his bedroom at the front of the house.

"Now the music will have to go into the music room." There was a second flight of stairs and she followed him, carefully holding a pile of old tattered music, up and round into an unexpectedly large attic room. What struck her was that after the bleakness and mess of the rest of the house, this was a well-ordered space with a desk in the dormer window, three instrument cases under the eaves – lute-like shapes. Music shelves to one side neatly stacked, and an ancient ornately carved wooden chair that looked like it dated back to Elizabethan times. The floor appeared to be made of old oak and there was a rich red Persian rug set in the middle. It was like stepping into another world, and Daniel could see the look of surprise on Melissa's face.

"I had all this done when I moved in. The floorboards are from a Tudor building that got knocked down to make space for car parking at one of the colleges, would you believe it? Still, I rescued them and fitted them myself."

So they went up and down stairs stacking the rest of the music neatly in a corner of the music room, then Daniel went off in search of the vacuum cleaner.

"Mrs Morgan does the house once a week, and I never get round to hoovering these days. It must be somewhere under the stairs." She heard a clattering from downstairs as she wandered round

149

her room in a daze, wondering how she would make it her own while she stayed. There was no wallpaper on the walls – it must have been stripped off with the intention of redecorating at some time in the distant past. It gave it a grimy look and she wondered if Daniel would stretch to a can of paint.

"Found it. Bag's nearly full. Can't find where I put the spares." He was out of breath and looked like he would just like to sit down after all their exertions. She was tired too, but she had to clean her room. The first step to making it her own.

"I'll make a cup of tea, unless... you want something stronger." She could tell from his voice that he was already thinking of opening another bottle of wine.

"Tea would be good." What about food? she wondered as she switched on the vacuum cleaner which made a high complaining noise. The bag was definitely full, but she managed to make a bit of a difference to the room.

A mug of tea was brought up and dumped by the door. "Fish and chips? There's a chippy just round the corner. Back in a sec."

So that's supper. She finished tidying the room as best she could, sat on the unmade bed and looked out of the window.

"So do you still live in South Oxford? You just came down here to give a lecture, you said."

"Yes, still at the same college. I could never move from that house after all we... after building that music room."

Why does he cover that up? All the work we did to make that house a home.

"Still got that deep red wall in my room?" I doubt it after the way I left, he must have redecorated.

"Oh yes, I couldn't paint over that." He blushes. "Is your... is James... OK? I mean what happened to... are you now with... him?"

"Yes." I see the disappointment flash across his face. There is

150

so much I haven't told him.

Chapter 18

"Why do I have to go back to school?"

"Why can't I just be allowed to drink whatever I want?"

Daniel and Melissa made a pact: she would go to the CFE and finish her education and he would curb his excessive drinking.

So many of the courses on offer looked attractive, but she had to do English Language before she could do anything else. On the literature front she was way ahead, she had read so much. And she continued to read after Daniel took her in. He got her a ticket for the Bodleian so she could read in peace without being thrown out by some officious manager, though she would probably have been left alone in her new M&S garb. Still, it was a privilege, and Melissa was constantly amazed that she could order whatever books she wanted, and they would be delivered to her at her quiet table. All she had to do was to promise not to burn the place down.

But they both knew that she needed to do something about her education. English Language! For all the reading, she could hardly put two sentences together. She was dyslexic. Spelling was appalling, but worse, she would lose confidence after a few sentences, grinding to a halt and wanting to harm herself. An expression of self-loathing after the fire, that a part of her that she thought she'd locked away for ever, delighted in. In a way it felt very similar to Daniel's excessive use of alcohol.

Why should they both want to hurt themselves when they had so much to give? She used that argument with him, he with her. So gradually, grindingly, they helped each other out of their respective holes – to treat themselves with respect and love.

His visits to the bottle dump became less frequent, and she began to manage paragraphs. These were heady times and they clung to each other like shipwrecked survivors. Their island made of music and words. The music sublime, the words... coming.

He would play to her of an evening after she had cooked him her latest version of Melissa-splodge. He sang to his lute, and though his voice was not beautiful, being used more as a tool for completing the music, the net effect was to pull her into his world. She loved his performances of Dowland, Cutting and so many other English lutenists. The songs were so often of unrequited love, and love at a distance. He lived this music and expressed it to her in a way that she knew was personal. His love for her that she couldn't return in the same way – the flower of a love that couldn't be consummated.

For her part she falteringly read him her essays, and he would help her improve the grammar and clarity of her writing, asking her questions to help her find her own words.

If she didn't work, or if he drank heavily, then that evening would have a heavy silence and would lose its magic. So they kept going, he got down to two glasses of wine a night and she managed to get a 'C' in English Language GCSE.

It was a magical time. They both knew it. The world was opening up to her now that she could write after a fashion, and his powers as a musician had returned and increased. He was doing more concerts and tours with his ensemble, and she was doing Environmental Studies at Brookes.

She wanted to contribute something to their household so she did waitressing. Tight black jeans, tight black t-shirt. Men looking at her, and the other girls – the sexy young waitresses. Were they the main attraction? Or was it really the food? Still, it meant that she could feel less beholden to Daniel, sweet Daniel.

 No, she wasn't being fair about the restaurant . The food was great, as was the ambience. She would have eaten there if she could have afforded it, and she wasn't interested in girls. Except as friends. She would go clubbing with them on a Friday night after work. The black t-shirt set. All eyes on them as they came through the door, but they would sit round a table like a bunch of gangsters, only allowing the odd privileged male to join them. The dancing was hypnotic, and they danced in a tight circle – forever desirable, forever unobtainable. Until...

James returns with Mistral and Monsoon bags. Forgetting myself I stand up and walk over to hug him. Daniel stares - surprised. I look down. There is the floor beneath my feet, but it's getting further away. I cling onto James, my firmness on this spinning planet, and the moment passes – he gently helps me back to my chair.

"Did I see what I thought I saw?" says a delighted Daniel.

"I don't know what happened."

"You moved without thinking about it," James says quietly, trying not to get too excited. "It must be like your speech, but..."

But how do I do that? It's like I have to catch myself unawares.

"I'm glad I was here and saw it." Daniel really does still love me. James looks anxious for a moment but I put my hand on his as he sits down beside me. I want to make love to him there and then. There is a huge difference between loving someone and being their lover, and although James and I have never crossed that threshold yet... we will.

Then she met Mike.

He was sitting in front of her in Environmental Studies Lecture Room 1.

Dark hair, strong masculine features as he turned his head – perfect profile, not pretty, not gawky. He wore glasses to work, but when he took them off to look round his blue eyes flashed with a brilliance as he caught hers. Standing up at the end of the lecture he revealed a perfect bum in tight jeans and she caught a couple of girls in her row giggling and nudging each other as they looked at him. He's mine, she thought then. Mine.

And so he was. It didn't take long – they met in the corridor after the lecture and he asked her if she'd like a coffee in the canteen. Just like that. Blam! Sussed girl in her twenties becomes a fledgling teenager. All eyes and blushes. All that work she had done carefully maintaining a platonic relationship with Daniel, with the world, gone in an instant of rushing chemicals. She just wanted to get her hands on him.

Mike had a bike and she mounted it behind him feeling the thrill of it between her legs as he revved the engine. He was her sex machine and they would make love when they got to his place in Cumnor. Perfect, perfect. They didn't go together like a porch and a rocking chair, they went together like the pistons of a steam engine. The power of brilliant sex overpowered everything else in her addled brain and she was his.

"I'm moving in with Mike." It was a painful conversation with Daniel. He looked so hurt. Those peaceful, creative evenings of music and words – all that they'd built together – would be finished. Gone. Like she'd slammed the door on them – on him.

"Thank you…" She couldn't say more at that point, the words just stuck in her throat.

"Are you sure… this is a good idea? This is so fast… you've only known him, what, three weeks." Daniel looked down trying to hide the tears. "You'll always be welcome back, you know."

That was it. She had to leave. Now. She wouldn't have this clinging parent figure holding her back any more. She had to go off and make babies with her man. Every fibre of her body screamed this.

"Goodbye."

Her few possessions – the clothes he'd bought her that winter day, and some other things she'd managed to afford herself, were packed in a couple of suitcases that Daniel lent her. She took one last look at her room which she had redecorated so carefully. It was suddenly much more difficult, a wrench to leave this place where she'd picked herself up. She sat on the stripped bed and looked out of the window at the park. A couple were kissing, there were children running and shouting. She couldn't look on any more – she had to go. Down the stairs, through the hall that she had redecorated and out of the front door that she had painted so carefully – four coats it took. A resonant blue.

She was gone.

Chapter 19

She had competition - his mother.

His mother Eva, the rich divorcee, had set him up in his nice flat in Cumnor, bought him his Ducati, paid for his beautiful clothes. He wanted for nothing - he was her boy.

Eva had dyed blond hair worn long, a beautiful figure, and a striking, almost masculine face. When they first met at Mike's flat, she took Melissa's hand in hers - perfectly manicured, slim-fingered, slightly bony.

"So glad to meet you."

"No you're not," she thought as Eva turned away to talk to her son about some detail to do with the flat, "she's leaving me out - pushing me out." To her, Melissa was just a shag-machine for Mike to keep him happy, keep him heterosexual (gay would be too bad for Mummy's boy) until she could find him the perfect bride, probably looking just like her. Well, she would just have to put up with Melissa for the moment, she wasn't going anywhere. It wasn't just sex they had, they told each other - it was love.

"I'd love to meet your family sometime," Eva said. She didn't mean it.

"You wouldn't," thought Melissa. "I have no family - they're either burnt to pieces or split up, and they certainly wouldn't want to meet you."

Money can do at least two things: if you're lucky it can help you relax about the world, and enjoy your time more without the constant fear of running out. Or it can make you never satisfied - always thinking you need more. Just that bit more to make you safe, just that bit more to control people and keep them where you want them. Eva was definitely the second type. Money was power and she couldn't get enough.

Mike saw through his mother and her games. He loved Melissa, or at least thought he did. He definitely wanted his freedom, but for that he would have to sacrifice all this cloying wealth. This mummy-cuddle money.

They had to curb their desire to just have sex all the time, and do some studying so that they could get good jobs and make some of their own money. They got through the first year of Environmental Studies and both realised it wasn't for them. Melissa's writing was slow and poor and Mike just couldn't read. Typical boy, he dragged himself through textbook after textbook not taking in anything. If they could have combined their abilities, his to write, hers to read, they'd have done alright. But as it was...

"I've been thinking about plumbing," Mike said one day over breakfast. "Loads of money and I could do a six-week course and get a qualification, and then get work. Everybody needs a plumber."

He was so gorgeous, so ever-optimistic. Melissa felt tears in her eyes as she leaned forward and held his arm.

"You don't have to abandon everything for me. You could still go for something more..."

"Academic?" he shrugged with a sad smile on his face. "I've never been much good at that, you know that."

"I love you Mike, I just don't want you to give up and settle for second best just for me."

"Mother wants me to do Film Studies. She thinks it will be good for me, less academic, but really she wants to keep me under her control."

"Is that what you want?"

"No... I just want to marry you and have a family and get away from her." He whispered this fiercely as though the walls would overhear him.

She heard him. "You want to marry me?"

"I do."

Silence.

She walked round the table and knelt on the floor to hug him round the waist. She couldn't speak, she buried her face in his chest and they stayed like that for a long time.

Chapter 20

However they broached it, Eva wasn't going to accept it. They took her power away and she screamed. She screamed in the flat, she screamed down the phone, she screamed to her friends, she screamed at their friends. They knew that they had to get away – her long sharp talons felt like they were deep in their shoulders. Their friends gave them support to start with, but then backed away, frightened by the ferocity of Eva's rage.

Chapter 21

I went down to St James's Infirmary
Saw my baby there
Stretched out on a long white table
So calm, so sweet, so sweet, so fair.

"I couldn't believe my eyes." James is flushed with emotion. We lie on the bed together looking up at the ceiling, our bodies relaxed after our first lovemaking. It hadn't been the greatest sex I'd ever had, my disability and lack of coordination didn't help, and James was shy and nervous. But it was the best. To have sex with someone I truly loved rather than thought I loved – that was very different.

"You walked over to me. Now we know you can do it. It will happen." He is so adamant, as though his life depended on it, not mine, and I feel a sudden unease as though we are sitting on a minefield and neither of us dare move for fear of mutual destruction.

"It's really important to you, you really need me to mend." I shift onto my side awkwardly to look directly into his eyes. I need to know something.

"Is it... is it to do with what happened before my accident? Alice's death? Am I... ?" I can't go on. His face changes as though a screen has come down behind his eyes.

"No, it's..." He is searching for the right words – words that would defend his position, hide his thoughts. "I feel responsible, so of course I want you to make the fullest recovery possible."

"But we've been over this before. It wasn't your fault, you couldn't have done anything to stop me running in front of you. It was entirely my doing, and there is no reason for you to keep blaming yourself. It's something else, isn't it?" God, you're the therapist, heal yourself, I say to myself as I lie back again to stare

165

up at the ceiling.

James remains silent.

"It's about Alice isn't it?" There it is. I've said it. Hit the mine, now wait for the explosion.

I expect him to get up and leave me now, but he turns over and buries his face in my chest and sobs.

Like the two of them, the years had run away. They still spoke to each other. The lovemaking was good – technically – but there was space where there should have been closeness, a silence that they tried to make comfortable by physicality. Time had worn down the façade of beauty of Mike's body, and hers, and they saw sinews, flesh, veins, bones, bloody organs beneath the surface of their once sun-kissed skins. To go back to that angel-air of mad love, chemicals boiling in a triumph of Eros: that was their longing – probably what kept them together.

And they were impoverished in another way. Down on the south coast, living wasn't cheap and Mike wasn't much good as a plumber. He took too long and often had to go back to correct a drip or a flood. His reputation went before him – 'Last-ditch Mick' he was known as. Melissa tried to resurrect her ability as a sculptor to make little figures and sell them, but it ended up costing her more money than it made. So she got some work as a proofreader but it was scant and irregular, and she was too slow for the better-paid jobs. Living the dream on the south coast was all very well but it wasn't a good place to get work unless you were willing to travel up to London every day, packed like a sardine.

Then, like a bright falling star it happened.

"I'm pregnant, I'm going to have your baby." They had waited so long without knowing it, and now it was happening. The smile on his face told her how much he wanted this. Had that been their trouble – an unadmitted feeling of failure on both sides? Had they really been longing for this all along, their own family, a reason

166

behind their lovemaking? She knew now that she had been, but Mike, he surprised her. He had never talked about his feelings on the subject - just shut down when she broached the idea of the family she had thought he wanted. Now he was alight.

"She's gone and I said I would always love her, and now I've fallen in love with you. I feel such a traitor."

"What happened?" I ask gently. "You've told me so little." I look gently into his eyes, but feel a bitterness inside. Am I just a second-best alternative to his true love?

He pulls away from me and shifts himself up into a sitting position, leaning against the pillows propped up at the bed head. I struggle to get into a position where I can look him full in the face. It's not easy for me but he makes no accommodation, caught in his own world.

"She'd just gone out shopping." It's as though he's delivering a well-rehearsed speech to an invisible audience. Tense, unemotional, dry as old bones. "She took the small car – we always used that for short trips. Used less petrol, save the planet we thought. There were roadworks. The light went red and the lorry in front stopped quickly. Alice stopped but the lorry behind her…" He can't go on for a moment, a catch in his throat shows how much feeling is being forced under control in order to get this out.

"The lorry behind her didn't stop and she was crushed between the two. No chance. No chance." He looks down, steeling himself.

I sense there's more.

A little life. Scarcely begun, but still there. It brought them together, and it brought her father back. She didn't know how he knew, but he rang one day out of the blue. Her father who deserted her. She should have felt angry. Put the phone down.

Walked away. But all she felt was joy and relief at hearing his voice.

"Dad, I'm going to have a baby." She could hear him gasp at the other end of the line.

"Mel, that's brilliant. My little Mel, you clever girl."

"Dad, I'm not your little girl any more, and you're going to be a granddad."

His voice went quiet, "It's so long since I've seen you. You were my little girl, and now you're..."

"Grown up."

There was a silence between them. On her side it was enmity mixed with longing. On his, just the longing.

"We must meet up." She could hear the guilt in his voice. Now the deserting father wanted to support his little girl.

They met in a greasy spoon café on the high street going down to the harbour. It had those high-backed benches with tables between, set like booths. They could talk privately, tucked up against the window with the melamine-topped table between them. A bit like being on a train.

She had forgotten how handsome he was. In his fifties now, but still slim and tall. A craggy face, well proportioned, topped with curly hair with a touch of grey in it. His blue eyes smiled out at her, and as he put his hand on hers, she noticed the chipped nails at the end of his muscular fingers. He had a gardener's hands. A long way from the civil service, and all that office work.

"Where are you living now?" she asked, not sure that she really wanted to know.

"I'm renting a cottage outside Folkestone. It's very convenient for work and it's got a kitchen garden where I grow my own vegetables."

Her very own dad, there in front of her after all this time. She swallowed her anger then, and lived for the moment.

"I missed you."

"Me too."

"I haven't told Mike that I'm meeting you. He would find it hard to understand. Sorry." Why did she say sorry? Did she want to protect herself – to protect this?

"I haven't seen your mother... since... I couldn't."

"How did you track me down?"

"I saw a card in the library. It said 'Melissa Smith – Proofreading'. It had your number and I took a chance."

"Yes, I kept my maiden name for professional work. But Dad, there must be hundreds of Melissa Smiths."

"I was all ready to make some excuse, it's not the first time, but... it was you. I didn't know you did that sort of thing. You were terrible at English at school. Art was your thing. Whatever happened?"

"I met a man in Oxford. He helped me out. He was kind."

Her dad looked down sadly, picked at his broken fingernails, and then looked up into her eyes. "Tell me," he said.

So she told him. She filled him in on her chequered history, watching the flickering emotions cross his face. The hard times with David, living on the streets in Oxford and being rescued by Daniel, meeting Mike and marrying him – she put a very positive slant on that part.

"What about you?" she asked.

So he told her he about how he had done various jobs after the lorry driving, picking up what he could, and was working as a gardener now looking after various private properties and second homes.

"I need to find a way of making more money. Now I've seen you, and I'm going to be a grandparent and all. It would be nice to have somewhere of my own where you could come and stay. Give you some support."

"About bloody time too," she thought, but she said: "But your gardening sounds so good, suits you so well. You look so well."

He shrugged his shoulders. "There's not enough money in it,

and I'm hopeless as a businessman. I should charge more, I know, but..."

He got up to go. He looked so sad. Meeting her had hurt him. Whatever peace he had found in his solitary life had gone now.

"Dad."

"Mel."

They hugged. It was almost harsh. Then he was gone.

James is crying again - his cold resolve broken down.

"I had to go and identify her. She was so crushed. They had cleaned her up as best they could. She was my Alice…" He sobs more and I touch him. His arm feels hard and cold – no response, caught in his grief.

"Those long white corridors, they just went on and on. Do you want a cup of tea? they said. A cup of tea? What good would that do? Do you want to talk to someone? Yes. Her!"

He is reliving all his pain, and I can't hold him. He swings his arms around in a rage nearly knocking me out of bed.

"James, James I'm here."

He looks at me, deranged for a moment. Blinks back more tears.

"I'm sorry. It's those corridors, horrible white corridors, I found myself back there, they went on for ever."

"I know, I know." And I do.

A little life in her. But something was wrong. Something was happening much too early. There was pain. There shouldn't be pain. There was blood. There shouldn't be blood. Mike was out. She couldn't get him on his mobile. She called the doctor. Stay still he said. She stayed still. The ambulance came. White doors closed her in. Nee-nah, nee-nah. Now she was in one, instead of thinking "poor sod" as she watched one go by.

She was wheeled down white corridors, endless white corridors.

170

Can they save my baby? Then, in a white, white room, on white, white sheets, there was her baby. Her baby, all bloody. That life that she was going to share. That beautiful little girl.

"Do you want to talk to someone?" they said. It had all been so quick. Mike was still out of contact. She needed someone. Dad. Phone Dad.

"Hello." His voice sounded clipped and there was noise. "Hello, I'm driving. Better make it quick."

"My baby," she sobbed, barely comprehensible. "I've lost my baby. She's dead, she's dead, she's dead."

"Oh... no..." She could hear his voice catching, she could see the tears in his eyes.

"Daddy, I need you."

There was a clunk, he'd dropped the phone, but she could hear the squeal of tyres and a big crunching noise.

"Oh shit, oh no." She could hear his voice in the distance, then the sound of a door being wrenched open. What was he driving? Was it a lorry? She never knew he'd gone back to lorry driving.

James is back in my arms. Somehow, awkwardly, I hold him. My precious love. He's back with me now, and I'm back with him, away from those terrible white corridors.

We just hug for a while. It's a bit painful for me, my body won't get into the right position. Then he says:

"He was on his mobile, the driver."

"What?" I let go and cover my face.

"His daughter had just lost her baby. I wanted to kill him, but... that good, good bit of me," James's voice is bitter now. "I had to understand. I didn't press charges, but the other part... the other part of me would like to see him hang!"

He is lost in his world of pain and anger again. He hasn't noticed me shaking, my face in my hands.

"Frank Smith, his name was. Bloody Frank Smith took my life

away."

At that moment I feel my life being taken away. I feel fear. Terrible fear. I had never guessed we could have this connection. I can't believe it. He's forgotten that my maiden name is Smith, he doesn't know about my lost baby. Like him and his loss, I have kept all that buried. Never wanted to talk about it. Wanted to escape from that dreadful time in my life. Now it has all caught up with me.

"James." I can't live with this. I take his hands and will him to look at me.

"James, I… do you love me?"

He looks lost for a moment, then nods his head.

"I need to tell you something." I should probably wait and tell him later, but I can't keep it in. "My father is called Frank Smith."

"So… there are probably lots of Frank Smiths, what's that got to do with anything?" He is angry at what he thinks is a flippant piece of information. "You've never even mentioned him before."

"I lost my baby." I can't go on, all this stuff that I've kept hidden. There's so much, now I've opened the cupboard door and it will all come spilling out.

James reaches out and holds me. He is the comforter now. It's so tempting just to stay silent in his arms, but that bit of me that insists on things being honest wrenches away from him.

"I told him," I wail. "I phoned him when he was driving and he had a crash. He was driving a lorry and crashed into someone and killed them. He went to prison. He didn't want to see me. I've haven't seen him since. I never knew he was driving lorries."

It's dawning on us, crashing in on us.

James is looking at me very steadily.

"So your father was Frank Smith." He's using all his powers as a psychotherapist to keep calm and clear. Almost disembodied.

172

Scary. "And you lost your baby. Why did you never tell me this before?" He is so ruthless. Where has my James gone?

"It was too... too..." I can't go on, I'm sobbing again. Scared. Hopeless.

"Did you know the name of the person he killed?"

Of course, that's why the name Alice made me uneasy. I buried it then – in hospital. I couldn't cope with it then. But Penhaligon? There was never a Penhaligon.

"I don't remember much about it. I was too... lost in my own stuff... I... It could have been Alice, but it definitely wasn't Penhaligon. Was it something like Cooper?" The sun is beginning to shine for me, relief floods in. It's a different accident – just an awful coincidence.

"It was her parents little joke," James says bitterly. "Alice Cooper. We were never married. We loved each other so much it didn't seem necessary... to marry. We were married in our souls, why did we need the Church or the law to add anything to that?"

Every word is a nail driven into me. He is so calm in his bitterness. He has forgotten me and is back with Alice.

"And to think I ran down the daughter of the man who killed my Alice."

He turns his back on me, gets out of bed and walks out of the room, a forlorn naked figure going beyond my reach.

Mike came and sat by her. Mute, hostile. How could you lose our baby? She read in his eyes. A brisk nurse came in – all business and light.

"Now your... partner's here, sunshine, let's see if we can get you up and going."

"He's not my partner," she muttered. "He's my husband and I'm not sunshine."

"Happens to lots of women, sunshine. You'll soon be as right as rain, and before you know it, there'll be the pitter-patter of tiny feet."

Later, she discovered that in all probability there would never be the 'pitter-patter of tiny feet'.

"Your miscarriage caused irreparable damage. The lining of your womb is very unstable and is likely to fall away once the pregnancy has reached a certain point." The specialist was blunt and to the point.

Why wasn't this picked up earlier during her checks? She had missed a couple of them, and the doctor always seemed in a hurry. Hassled, hair-falling-out type. Melissa was afraid to ask questions. Didn't want to be a nuisance.

So that was it.

Her baby was torn out of her hands, her father was in jail, her husband was losing interest. Her mother? Could she go back there? Her mother came to visit her one day. Blast of trumpets! She just talked about herself, and about Melissa's dead brothers. If she'd had a shotgun Melissa might have put her mother out of her misery. But fortunately there was the door, and she showed it to her, and her mother went through it.

Then the mystery.

Someone paid for Melissa to go to Australia.

At the time, she was so distressed she just accepted it and went, but on her return she never found out. Should have tried harder, but she guessed that her benefactor wished to remain unknown. She wondered though: was it Daniel? Or even her dad from prison?

It certainly wasn't Mike, though he was glad to see the back of her for a month. When she returned she felt a subtle shift in his attitude to her. He seemed secretive and she guessed he'd been using his plumbing to please some housewife or other. He was getting more work now, so he said. Sometimes he had to work late – probably in somebody else's bed, certainly not in hers. Their lovelife had died with the baby, and she knew then that it had simply been chemical. The extraordinary thing was how long the chemistry had lasted. Scientists would have had a field day with them proving that love was no more than an exchange of molecules or whatever.

Then the mother-in-law from hell returned. Melissa even wondered if Eva had paid for her Australian trip to get her out of the way. Mike's mummy came back and scooped him up and took him away. And that was that. No more sullen silences, no more slammed doors, no more being woken in the middle of the night. No more lonely marriage. And Melissa packed the boxes, never guessing what would happen next.

Flight

Chapter 22

"Paragliding? Isn't that very dangerous?" The thought of it makes me shiver – all that way to fall to the ground.

"I'm going to try it. I need a sport. It's only a couple of days. I need..."

To get away, I think.

"It's a challenge, I know. But I'll be alright. They're very good teachers and it's just the South Downs."

"But, but..." I trail off. I can't think what to say. He is at one remove from me now. Polite. Generous even, but in a different dimension. I am not forgiven for what my father did, and he won't talk about it. Alice has come back into his life and knocked me out. Dead Alice.

"Look, I've got to go. You'll be alright, there's food in the fridge. You're so much more mobile now... you'll be alright."

I wish he wouldn't say that. How can I be alright after what happened?

Our first lovemaking...

The end.

I feel the tears start. Until this moment I had felt cold, stunned, but now the sobs are rising in my chest. I can't control it. I put my head in my hands and weep.

"You'll be alright." He puts his hand on my shoulder for a fleeting moment, and then turns and leaves the room. I hear the front door close, the sound of the car door opening and closing, the engine starting up, the sound of the car fading, and he is gone.

I don't know how long I sit there, cold disbelief turning my body to stone. The sobbing and shaking has stopped but I am stuck, caught in a change of wind, face frozen.

It's been a week since our terrible discovery. A week of my hoping he would come back to me. He is a psychotherapist, I thought. He will reflect, get through it, realise that he must move on. Gentle James, lovely James. He will come back. Psychotherapist heal thyself. Except he doesn't. I don't understand how he manages to work – help other people in their lives when his is so screwed up. But that's the thing about psychotherapy, the system works as long as the therapist doesn't bring himself and his issues into the room. It's what the patient brings to the room that matters. If only he could sit there in his own room and be his own therapist and see what he's doing. But he can't and we're stuck.

We have functioned for a week. He has been gentle, has made sure I get to my physio. He has looked out for me in a physical way. I have been able to get around the house more easily, without using the wheelchair. I have even been able to cook a little, taking care not to spill things on myself. But inside it has been a desert, a cold, cold place. I want to shout,

"IT'S NOT MY FAULT MY FATHER KILLED FUCKING ALICE!"

I want to smash things – throw plates and glasses on the floor. Get her photo that has looked at me so enigmatically from the sittingroom mantelpiece, and break the frame, tear the picture to shreds. Alice, Alice, Alice. If you weren't dead I would never have found my love, my James. So go away now. Leave us alone. Stop haunting us. We both need to move on in the living world. You're dead. We're alive. So GO AWAY!

All my ranting inside did no good. James couldn't hear me. Alice couldn't hear me. I didn't dare let anyone hear these thoughts, but kept them to myself. I nearly spilled out my feelings to Georgie during my physio session but she was so blown away by my sudden improvement. She didn't see me – she saw my body. "It's a miracle," she said. "All your hard work, all James's support has paid off."

That support, that so-needed person, where's that support now?

It was she, not James who contacted Mark the neurologist. "Well done, well done!" he said, and then broke into a ramble of incomprehensible jargon, the gist being the wonders of the brain. Where are the wonders of my heart?

I am untouchable. Nobody wants to touch me. But honestly, for all the cold rage flowing through my veins, there is a warm receptive heart beating there. Waiting for someone to reach out to me. Waiting for James.

But now he's gone.

Finally, after what seems like hours, I decide to move. I need to do something. I can't stay like this for ever.

I lift myself out of my chair and stand up. I can walk, I remember. But my legs have forgotten. They are weak and they wobble uncontrollably, and I sit down again with a bump. I must just be stiff. I rub my legs, wriggle my bottom in the chair to get movement back into my muscles. Flex my feet, move my legs up, down. Side to side.

Right, that's better. Now stand up.

I can't. It's just the same, my legs wobble uncontrollably and I sit down again with a bump.

After all the tears and anger I begin to feel panic. I really am stuck. I am stuck in this chair. Once more, the floor seems a long way away. All that precious ground that I had gained has gone and I'm back with my terror of falling. My head begins to spin, I feel sick. I can't stay here all day. I have to eat, I have to pee, I have to shit.

My chair is an upright one with arms, but I have pushed it back away from the table where we had our breakfast. The things are still there on the table. Cold toast, crumby butter, an open pot of yogurt, two empty mugs. All on a nice white linen tablecloth.

It's out of my reach, but if I could just get up and lean towards it, maybe I could use the table to support myself and get to the wall. Once I've got to the wall, I can get anywhere in the house – eventually.

I ease myself cautiously out of the chair, my legs wobbling, my head swimming, and I make a lunge for the table. But my legs don't support me even long enough for that, and I grab at the tablecloth as I fall to the floor. Something hard hits me on the head. It's my mug, the one James bought for me. I see it as it hits the floor and bounces – it doesn't break. I see the pretty tree painted on it. I remember the childish delight I had when he gave it to me. I pick it up, my head is swimming still and something hurts, and I hurl it with all my might at the wall. It smashes sending sharp bits of bone china all over the floor. The floor that I will have to crawl on if I'm going to get anywhere.

I just lie there for a while, trying to gather my wits. What am I trying to do? I've got to move. I need to get to the bathroom to clean my teeth. I'll need a pee soon as well. In fact... no don't think about it.

So this is it. I must crawl round the house. I get up from my side where I have fallen and find that my left wrist is really painful. It must have taken my weight when I fell grabbing the tablecloth with my right hand. I don't think it's broken, just sprained. But I can't put my weight on it. Instead I use my left elbow, and with my right hand flat on the floor I manage to slide along on my left side. It is painful, I must have bruised my left hip in the fall, and with my sudden increased lack of coordination it is slow going. I pull myself through the debris of my smashed mug, trying not to cut my hand on the tiny shards, and make my way to the door. I drag my body slowly down the corridor towards the downstairs bathroom that he created specially for me. My need to pee has become stronger now, I am desperate to hold on. Not to let myself down. For whom? I wonder. I turn through the doorway into the bathroom and reach up for the grab-rail to the side of the toilet. I get myself up into a kneeling position facing the bowl, but still have to work out how to turn round. My head is spinning again and I feel sick. I grab the loo seat and gradually shift my way round so that I can get hold of the rail on the right hand side and pull myself up. I manage to get up into a sitting position perched on the edge of the loo seat, and I try to take my trousers down with my good hand, but it's too late. Urine streams down my legs and onto the floor. In my heightened state of anxiety it smells strong, I feel like I have flooded the bathroom.

Humiliated. In pain. Abandoned.

I look above the sink beside me to the bathroom cupboard. There are sleeping pills in there. I needed them once, and I need them now. There are lots left over. We should have thrown them away weeks ago, but they are still there. I can reach the cupboard door with my left hand. My injured wrist hurts madly as I try to open the door, but I am determined now. This is the way to go. I can't live life without James. I can't bear the thought of my condition getting worse, and it seems like I am back at square one today. Take the pills. Go to sleep. Finish it now. I hope it hurts him too. He has so hurt me, and I realise how angry I am with him. I can't ever forgive him for what he's done. Tears of fury make it difficult to see and find the packets of sleeping pills. I grab at the pile, dropping two packets into the basin, and there they are, the sleeping death.

Now I need water to wash them down and I reach out to pick up my plastic tooth mug from the side of the wash basin, pouring out my toothbrush and paste into the bowl and clumsily filling the mug with water. Ugh, it's warm from the wrong tap and there is a flavour of mint from my bits of toothpaste stuck to the side of the mug. I had meant to clean it but never got round to it. Too late now.

I shovel the hastily pressed-out pills into my mouth and take a gulp of water, nearly gagging on the warm sweet minty fluid. More in, more water down. Then I take the soggy packets from the basin and press the pills out of them as well. Cold water this time, less minty. Better.

That's all I can find and I sit and wait.

I sit there for a long time, waiting to feel the effects. Then as I start to get drowsy, I realise I've left it too late to get down on the floor in any controlled fashion. My head starts spinning and I see the lino with its puddle of urine coming up towards me. I fall hard onto my injured wrist, jarring it again, the pain surging through me. I feel the damp shame of my failure soak into my clothes. I see the walk-in shower where James so carefully bathed me, and I lose consciousness.

Chapter 23

I'm running through trees. There is fear in my blood and I don't know whether I'm running after something I desperately need, or away from something that I desperately want to escape from. I am running fast with a feeling of strange joy – I feel so alive, though somewhere in my memory, I am dying. The trees crowd in on every side. It is a deep forest. The light penetrates in places, but there is a lot of darkness surrounding me. There is something odd happening to my bones – they feel lighter, thinner. Then they begin to change shape. I feel my skin stretch, and my muscles pulled. I crash into a tree on my left and see blood running down my arm. I keep running but as I look, to my horror I see something dark and matted grow out of my skin where I have cut myself. My arm is lengthening – stretching out and down and it puts me off balance and I crash into another tree, on my right this time. The same is happening to my right arm, but I'm still running. Faster if anything. I am getting lighter and despite the pain of my lacerated skin, movement is becoming more effortless.

Then something happens to my mouth. I can feel my nose and lips being drawn forwards, and a terrible pain in my teeth. Everything is grinding and stretching, pulling out of shape. The shapes of the trees flash past in a blur. My perception is changing. My clarity of vision is narrowing and sharpening, as though I'm looking through binoculars. In the distance I can see a light, and I'm speeding towards it ever faster. I open my mouth and let out a hoarse cry. It sounds strange and alien to my ears, and when I try to move my lips to speak I find that they are hard, fixed and rigid. I can only make this strange hoarse sound. Then my stomach starts to feel too full as though I am going to burst with its heavy contents. Much too heavy for me now. I open my mouth, and instead of my weird sound, out pours a projectile vomit of bones, flesh, organs. My old insides are being rejected, and a new order is inside me. Lighter, simpler.

My legs suddenly give way. I can't feel the ground any more. I look at my arms and they are covered in black feathers. The pain in them has gone now, and instead there is a strange electricity. The feathers grow and stretch out and I have wings. My legs are short and useless for running, but I haven't fallen. By some miracle my wings are supporting me and my legs are off the ground. I'm heading for the light, and with a shock I find I'm out of the trees, the ground falls away and I'm looking down a mile to jagged pink rocks and a distant river.

Then I begin to fall. Fear has made me rigid. I am not a flyer, I am a human being, and I'm not meant to jump off the edge of cliffs into a canyon. I will die, crushed by my own weight as I hit the distant ground at a huge velocity. But I'm not falling like a stone. My wings are flapping like wet rags as I spiral down, but surely this is not a human fall. Humans don't have wings.

"Wake up," says a familiar voice. That Aussie voice which helped me across a bridge is back. "Be a bird. You've got wings, haven't you? Fly."

I test my wing muscles. In spite of the speed at which I am travelling downwards, I can shape my wings with extreme effort. Instead of flapping about uselessly I can hold them in some kind of shape. The descent stops abruptly and I find myself hurled upside down. I flap uselessly for a moment feeling completely out of control, but manage to get myself the right way up again. I feel very precarious, floating up so high with just these wings to support me. It feels like the slightest change in angle will cause me to flip and lose control. And I do so a number of times before I get the hang of it. My fear is receding, except there is a wild natural awareness of danger that I suspect is part of being what I am now. I feel a fierce joy as I circle above this great space. The air holds me up, and every now and then a thermal pushes me higher - I can feel the warm air and something in me responds to it naturally.

186

"Wow, that was some trick!" I hear this in my head at the same time as I am aware of a large black bird gliding next to me making a strange duck-like noise.

"That wasn't a trick. I'm just working out how to fly." I find I'm making the same caw-caw quack-quack noise but hearing my words in my head. The concentration involved in doing this puts me off my newly-attained balance and I go into another flappy tumble, but this time manage to right myself without doing more than one somersault.

"Hey man, you learning to fly in one of the world's premium surfing spaces, and you a full-grown raven. You crazy or something?" He sounds like a he. I don't know how you tell, but I sense it.

"I was something else before and I just turned into a bird without knowing what was going on."

"One of the magical sisterhood, eh?" He shrugs his shoulders and glides effortlessly away and up. I have to flap furiously to catch up with him.

"What do you mean?" I gasp.

He doesn't reply, but just goes into a dive, aiming for the canyon floor. I watch anxiously as he heads for certain death, dropping like a stone. Then he just effortlessly comes out of his dive, spreads his wings catching a thermal and is soon a dot heading across the canyon.

So I'm a raven. Didn't I hear somewhere that they were the best flyers of all? Certainly the most intelligent. How does so much brain get packed into such a small space? Interesting that I can only vaguely remember what I did before I became a bird. Something about eating the wrong stuff. Well, I'll have to be more vigilant. I am hungry now, I realise. But what do I eat? I look back at the edge of the canyon from which I emerged, but all I can see is forest and trees. Something in my mind says "people". But surely I don't eat people. I glide along the edge of the canyon – flying near the rim is very easy as the warm air from below hits the wall of the canyon and bounces up like a wave, supporting me.

It isn't long before I see the trees pull away from the edge and buildings appear. They are large wooden buildings, with garishly-painted signs on them. There are plenty of people about, going in and out of them. Something tells me there is food around. I can smell it all over the place. It seems to be coming from small bins, placed near the buildings for people to put food into. I have a vague memory of having looked in these sort of bins in my human past, when I was hungry, though it feels a rather unsavoury memory. These bins smell different. They are brimming with delicious food kindly put there for my convenience.

I choose a bin that's on its own, away from the crowds of people, and practise my first landing. It doesn't go well, I don't quite know where my feet are, and my wings, which have just got used to gliding, flap in a most ungainly manner. I realise too late that being a big bird close to the ground is harder work than being, say, a sparrow, and I crash head first into the bin, my beak getting stuck in the side of a plastic bottle. I scramble and flap back out of the bin, shaking my head furiously from side to side to get rid the bottle, and perched precariously on the edge, I send it clattering across the ground. So much for a discreet feed.

A group of humans have been attracted by the noise and they point at me, laughing and getting black metal objects out of their clothes.

"What a clown!" I hear one say. "Do you think it will do the trick for us again? I'd love to have it on camera."

Clown? I'll show them. I pick at a meaty ball and hold onto it while I try to take off and eat it in private. I overbalance and crash into the wall onto which the bin is attached, dropping most of my treasure in the process. There are gales of laughter as I manage to take off with a clumsy flap of my wings.

"What a clown!" rings in my ears as I carry my food off to a safe place in the trees away from my persecutors. I greedily settle down to eat what's left in my beak, but then comes the next surprise. It just tastes of dust. Dry. Nothing. I can't eat it and I spit it out. It must be the wrong sort of food – processed human muck. I need real meat.

I take off, with more control this time, and gain height to see what is around. I am amazed by my eyesight. I can see for miles. Everything is so clear – such good quality. If I was a camera I would be the best ever made. In the distance, something attracts my attention. I smell blood. "Meat," says my raven-brain. Carrion. Something dead that I can eat. I fly over the trees to a clearing, and there, spread out before me for my delight, is a half-eaten deer. Tender bits of flesh are exposed; I can hardly wait and I swoop down and land on the carcass, ready for a feast.

"Not so fast," a voice says behind me, and I look round to see a huge vulture waddling towards me, its sharp curved beak open ready to slash at me if I don't move. "This is for me and my buddies. Now scram!" I see other large shapes descending and know I am outnumbered, but I still take a quick slice of the booty in my mouth, dodging the bigger birds as they make for me, talons outstretched.

I'm up and away, catching the air currents, a much better flyer than the clumsy old vultures. And I'm just a beginner.

I find a spot to enjoy my stolen booty. Tear it up, wolf it down.

Dust. It just tastes of dust. I spit it out, coughing and spluttering. If I can't eat food, how am I going to stay alive?

Then I remember the surfing raven's words – 'magical sisterhood'. Where have I come from? I wasn't born a raven. I did something, ate something wrong, and here I am.

I am a spirit bird. Didn't the tribes of North America talk about birds in this way? And where am I? This has got to be the Grand Canyon, home to many tribes. Hualapai, Havasupai, Navajo, Paiute, Hopi, and Zuni.

So I'm a spirit bird. I'm hungry but can't eat. This hunger is for

189

something else and I must search the world for it. I've been given eyes and wings, and a natural intelligence. So I must stop playing the clown, the child, and think.

"Up, up," I think and my wings obey me. A slight flap and I catch the rising air current and am gliding up high above the trees to get a view of the Grand Canyon. The Colorado River shines far below me, going west to the sea, but I must go east. My instinct tells me this. I must fly east across this great land using every good current I can find. So I enter that bed of air and glide along the south rim following the canyon as it goes north and east. Every now and then a surfer-raven whizzes past me going down to do that amazing trick of gathering speed and shooting across the ten miles to the north rim. But I am a spirit bird and I am above such things.

"Oh go on," says a voice in my head. "You'll never get another chance." So I throw caution to the winds, literally, and dive. I pull my wings in tight. "Ha Jonathan Livingstone, the ravens got there first. We've been doing this for centuries." My downward velocity is screaming in my ears. I begin to wonder if a spirit bird can die – crashing into the hard rock of the valley floor. "Don't think about it – do it," says that voice in my head. I keep my nerve, and let my body work it out. A slight increase in wingspan, and then spread full out and catch that wave of air. I have dropped the best part of a mile in thirty seconds, and the speed and energy attained, shoot me out across the canyon in a spirit-lifting moment. This is flying! I am going so fast that I can flip over onto my back and fly upside down looking into the sun. I roll and roll, enjoying the sensation and then speed across the great space looking down at towers of rock carved into magical shapes by time. This is a truly spiritual place and I feed on it like a whale on plankton, swallowing up the goodness to prepare for my journey north and east.

The north rim of the canyon is higher and colder than the south and has a wilder beauty. I follow my route looking at green meadows to the north and arid desert to the south. Forest and rock take over and I am leaving the Grand Canyon to fly above the river valley up to Glen Canyon and the canyon lands.

Chapter 24

With all this beauty below me, I forget how hungry I am.

I want to see the great rocky edifices of Monument Valley and so I take a turn south and travel a while until I am looking over a bizarre landscape to huge and impossible square lumps of rock towering above the plain below. Many lost worlds here, and I become lost myself in the experience of flying alongside the great cliffs, carving up in my mind this beauty of hewn colour and space. I am so swallowed up in this lesson of time, water and landscape that when the hunger kicks in I feel like I'm going to die.

"Get back on the track," a voice says inside me. "North and east or you will cease to exist." The pain is terrible. It drives me back onto my route, and as I obey my instinct, the pain gets less until it goes back to the dull ache reminding me of how empty I am. I am alone too. Since my encounters in the Grand Canyon I have met no more birds – almost as if I don't exist in their world and they don't exist in mine. My inner navigation system tells me to fly higher, going up into the clouds and above them like an aeroplane.

As a raven, I am instinctively wary of planes. When you watch them from ground level they look slow in comparison to how they actually are up in this thin air. Five hundred miles an hour is a ridiculous speed close to, I realise as one of these silver giants appears and disappears with a deafening roar of air and jet fuel. Get too close and that monster would swallow me up, ejecting me out again in impossibly small pieces. I am a spirit bird, so I don't know if this would happen to me, but I'm not about to find out. I am in their territory, so I use all my raven awareness and eyesight to keep out of their way. No sensible bird would be up here. Certainly no bird that needed to eat.

But this high route suits my mission. I fly fast and directly without distraction, away from storms, and admittedly away from thermals. But thermals work both ways. You can follow them for ease of flying, but they can take you right off course, and I can't go off course, so they are as much a hindrance as a help.

Lonely and cold, but fast and direct, I plough this eerie landscape over clouds far above land, until I sense the sea below me. I have been high above the clouds for so long that I have lost track of time, of day and night. It has been a cold meditation – no comfort, just driving force and concentration, feeling the hunger pulling me on. Perhaps from mind-numbing boredom, or a wish to be in contact with my route, I am drawn down below cloud level to fly above the heaving sea.

At first it looks blue and enticing. A jolly jaunt across the rolling main. But as I get closer the colour changes to green flecked with white and I sense the wild sea. The waves are huge and powerful, surging relentlessly across this seemingly infinite mass of water. Concealed beneath them are secrets that I shall never find out. There is food down there and mad loons dive into these surging waters, coming out again miraculously with a burden of fish. They see me with their wild red eyes but ignore me, probably wondering what this insane raven is doing flying far away from food and land. Intent upon their cold feast they dive ceaselessly, coming up again and again with enough food to feed thousands. They can see what I can't – a great shoal down below the surface of the sea.

I fly on leaving them to their harvest, skimming the surf-topped waves. My direction is unerring, taking a direct route north-east across what must be the Atlantic away from the coast of Canada.

I feel a subtle shift in wind and air pressure. This is a warning. There is a great force coming my way. There are no sea birds about now and the skies are darkening. A storm is coming up from the south and I see it on the horizon, a dark mass coming towards me at incredible speed. I can't avoid this. I should have stayed above the clouds but now it is too late. The first outriders strike me, buffeting me northwards. Bullies pushing me off course with ever

194

increasing intensity. It is all I can do to stay up in the air, and I use all my skills, both innate and recently learnt, to deal with this mass of unthinking energy.

Hah! I am a raven. The greatest of flyers. I can say that as much as I like but the wind is my world, and when it chooses to be this strong no bird can resist it. I am blown north, carried by the wind, and starvation sets in. The pain would be even worse if it wasn't for the immense hard work I have to do just to keep alive. If I relax my guard for a moment I will be turned into an out-of-control ball of feathers somersaulting into the waves.

The battering goes on and on, and I'm being driven to my death. I am getting weaker with starvation, but inside I want to live. I want to make my journey. I know it's important, essential, the meaning of my life. All the feelings of bad luck, strife, love, emptiness, questions, and unfinished business, come back to me as I struggle to stay alive, giving me unexpected strength, and I battle on against the howling forces that mindlessly seek to destroy me.

More suddenly than it came, it's gone.

I am drifting above the disturbed sea. In the distance I see a white line and my oversensitive ears can hear the sound of breakers. It must be land on the horizon. The storm has blown me so off course that I can't tell what it is that I'm heading for – what land lies ahead. But my inner compass tells me that at least I am flying in the right direction again. The hunger pangs are bad, but are getting less as I fly towards the white strip of land. I am not going fast as I am so weakened by wind and hunger, but steadily the white line gets closer, and the sound of crashing breakers louder.

As I get nearer I see that the white line is much higher than it looked at a distance. White cliffs confront me, but they are not the chalk cliffs of Dover. They stretch in a vast band from left to right as far as the eye can see, and they are made of ice. Their height, too, is formidable. A white barrier slicing into the sea, cutting into the swirling maelstrom beneath me. Still, solid ice.

The crash of the waves against this great wall is deafening now. I must climb if I'm going to avoid the spray which shoots up hundreds of feet. But I have little strength left and it feels like I'm being dragged down to sea level by the freezing cold air coming off the cliffs. No friendly canyon thermals here. I struggle up against cold draughts, feeling the spray of the waves making my feathers wet and heavy, and as I get nearer to the giant cliffs I hear a cracking sound. Not the constant crash and boom of the breakers, but a deeper sound - the sound of heaven and earth being torn apart, the groaning of tortured giants. Then to my horror the cliff starts falling towards me – a wall of solid crushing ice. I am too late and too low to avoid it and I fly blindly, expecting to be pulled down and crushed under its huge weight. All around me I hear the shrieks and groans of splitting ice, reluctantly breaking up for the first time in a million years.

Deaf, blind, I feel nothing. No pain. A white cloud bears me up and up. It is cold, very cold. Opening my eyes I look down. The cliff wall is descending into the sea – collapsing on itself right in front of me, and sending up a huge cloud of tiny ice particles. This is what is bearing me up. Like cold smoke it pushes me up and over the top onto this frozen land. I ride the ice cloud in a blaze of light, like God's hand has pulled me up. "You haven't finished," I hear that Aussie voice say.

Then all is silence.

I glide above a white landscape, stretching out as far as I can see – the sun making it blaze with cold light. The wind has dropped after its efforts during the storm, and the crash of descending ice and sea breakers is hidden by the sharp edge of this new world. There is nothing to make any sound. No life, nothing moves, and the wind is still. If I hadn't heard that voice I would wonder if I was actually dead, and this was my dead-flight-world.

But my raven-mind knows that this is Greenland, and that this vast expanse of ice on rock will go on for hundreds of miles. My hunger is back too, searing pain with nothing to distract me – another sign that I am still alive and on my journey. I seem to float above this stillness, but slowly, gently, a breeze starts up, pushing me on my course. At first it is a high hissing sound, it feels like it's in my head, a bit like tinnitus. But I feel the gentle push of the infant air current, and I know that it is the start of something big. A wind that pushes me across the world.

My tiredness is extreme and I am cold too, but the air is pushing me now and I spread my wings out and feel the sun on them. Solar energy – my black feathers soak it up and the warmth feeds me as I fly through this lonely landscape. It seems at times that I am asleep, but I dream of the same thing – this endless white. When I wake it is just the same, so I am never sure what is sleep and what is not. The sound of the wind increases gradually, and begins to howl and moan – that horror-house sound that will make you scared on a lonely moor. But here it is my friend, pushing me on with increasing speed, guiding me to my destination. That, and my hunger which is ever-present.

I lose track of time in my sleeping-waking world. Ever the same. Seemingly unending. Perhaps this is peace. But not for ever – the restless mind must have something to feed on. If this went on for ever it would kill my mind – drive me to a still madness. So it is a shock, but a welcome one when I come to the end of this white land and spy the sea surging in front of me.

Chapter 25

They're back. Mad red eyes, sharp pointed beaks. Their bulging bodies made sleek for the suicidal dive. Loons surround me, ignoring me completely in their death-defying search for food. They are masters of these cold seas, diving so deep that they should be swallowed up by the powerful ocean, but always rising like watery phoenixes with a fresh burden of fish.

I have to work hard over these choppy seas, keeping a weather eye out for another storm. I could gain altitude and fly in higher safety, but the activity of these birds and others keeps me low. Although they ignore me, I like their company. It makes me feel alive after my long sleep-glide over Greenland. Hunger drives me south-east now, the main wind currents would carry me directly south so I must work to get to Iceland.

No storms come my way, and it is sooner than I expect when I spy Iceland in the distance with my binocular vision courtesy of Raven Inc. Curiously, as I come to accept my raven-ness and enjoy it, I feel my human-ness coming back too. Memories of my life and what I am going back to, enter this tiny brain of mine. There is limited space inside me, but essential things like people and places are beginning to find their way back in.

Iceland is a play park for us birds who have braved the Arctic. The warm springs and geysers provide food and welcome relief for thousands of birds. No good to me though. I must travel on now southwards to the Shetlands, Orkneys, and on to the land that is my home.

Reluctantly leaving the Iceland haven, I work my way across the seas to the Shetlands. I hope for rest here, but no chance. Apart from the hunger that drives me on, there is a menace that many birds fall foul of. A sudden flash of something brown and white above me – I am the target of speed and aggression. This bird is not ignoring me like the others but is intent on my destruction. I avoid its first lunge, but it leaves me flapping to regain balance as another murderous seabird dives at me. This one catches a wing and I feel pain. Me, the spirit bird, the raven, caught in a storm of large killer birds. I must think quickly. "Skuas," a voice says in my head. "Get out quick." They will attack anything. It could be for food or to protect their young, but they will show no mercy, these pirates.

I do the opposite of the expected, and instead of being driven down, I head straight up and at the next bird. It doesn't flinch but makes straight for me. I hold my course until the last split second, and then, with a flick of my wings, skim past it. Too large to turn, it misses me and I fly up till I am well above the mobbing skuas.

My wing is hurting – no bones broken but some feather damage. I will live with the pain, at least I am alive and going south. As I fly on, I begin to realise something. I had been ignored by other birds for so long that I thought I must be a ghost. But these pirates spotted me.

And another thing – I am beginning to hear voices. They are faint at the moment, but the farther south I fly, the louder they get. Snatches of conversation, mostly not making much sense:

"Lost it... go north... windy here... ah food... get off my... babies... for this time of year..."

This babble goes on inside my head, but I can't make out where it's coming from. Perhaps I'm losing my mind – too much information for such a small brain. The babble is getting steadily louder. All I can see is the sea below me, so where is this all coming from?

Then I spot a dark object on the horizon. It is moving across the sea at a snail's pace. A ship. As I get closer I see the size of it. It looks half a mile long, black and belching smoke.

"My space... my space... my space... my space...," a repetitive call comes up from its stern, and I see a flock of seagulls and realise it is their voices I hear in my head. They are whirling around

200

jostling for position as rubbish is chucked into the sea from the ship. The cardboard boxes and food waste land behind the ship's huge stern, and the gulls go silent, so intent are they on scavenging their meals. I can feel the tension as they dive again and again searching for morsels. Fish and chips, burgers in baps, unspeakable green sludge. All this is their goal. I look down in disgust, then I remember my foraging at the Grand Canyon, and remember too the lure of human cast-off food.

The voices start up again: "Mine...no mine... get out of it... that's my sausage... nothing in this box...," and so on. The flock bickers over the remains after their first concentrated dive for food.

I hover round the ship. It must be a supertanker. Black and depressing, it makes its slow endless journey round the world. There is a great feeling of sadness coming from the towering block that makes the living quarters at the back end of this long, long sea monster. I sense oil, and it's almost overpowering, but the sadness seeps out and up into the air. A sense of loss, of missing loved ones, of longing, of desperate need to get off this endless circling of the globe. I fly above the living quarters lost in this depression. Caught up in the melancholy that runs this huge monster ship.

I realise that this reflects my mood too. My sense of loss, of missing someone, and suddenly I don't want to be there any more. I want to go south to my homelands, to find... whatever it is I am starving for.

I leave the squabbling chatter of the gulls and the melancholy thoughts of the men, and fly south to find land.

The babble of small voices attracts my attention, and there below me must be the Orkneys. No skuas here that I can see. Just lots of smaller birds wading on the shore. Very noisy they are too.

"Oyster there... give over... ow... who do you... my go... tum-te-tum... wave, look out..."

Oyster catchers dance and prance in the shallows, happily picking at the seafood so generously provided by nature.

Then one spies me: "Raven... raven, raven, raven, RAVEN!" the cry is taken up and panic spreads. Am I really that dangerous?

Then I spot something really dangerous out of the corner of my eye. So do they: "Skua, skua, skua, SKUA!" Everybody scatters as the great pirates dive with murderous intent. Where did they come from? I head up and away from the danger. I must reach the mainland now. Get away from these wild seas and over my own land.

The sounds of the raid recede, and I hear the fragmented domestic sounds of small birds going about their business. I keep my distance, flying high and heading south across the last small band of sea.

Chapter 26

Sea breezes sweep the coast, and I cross them – travelling southwards. It's quieter on the mainland. My hunger is less now, though my mind is beginning to focus on my goal. The reason I am here. There are people I must find, I sense two of them. There is a longing and an urgency lodged somewhere in my consciousness. But the land I am in swallows up my thoughts – takes my mind on another journey as I turn southwards.

Out of the rugged plains, mountains.

Each one to be savoured, explored.

So good to be with these massive shapes, flying low. Experiencing them without the sweat and toil of having to scramble up their steep sides on clumsy human legs.

An unusual part, this northern extreme. Not ranges of mountains as further south and west, but individuals rising out of the moorlands. Their beauty visible on all sides.

I zig-zag my way southwards, taking in lochs and forests. There is very little babble of birds here, and as night falls the sound of bellowing red deer: "Gather round, gather round, you are my herd. Keep safe."

Darkness falls for the first time on my long flight. I have followed the light, or slept on the wing, but now I experience the night.

Silently, black on black I course the highlands. The constant chatter of bird-thoughts is silent now. The occasional ghostly owl passes by, only making sound to frighten prey. One looms out at me unexpectedly, its huge eyes staring balefully, pale and luminous. "Raven," is all it says as it glides on, dismissing our encounter as a distraction from its hunting.

I pass over a group of bats hunting moths. They sound like recorded conversation being played backwards. Oddly eerie and alien, I can't understand a word.

Moving fast now, a dark shape skimming across the moon. My

hunger is less urgent, but more distinct. Like I am nearer the food that I need to eat.

Dawn breaks, and with it a cacophony – so many voices at once from the small birds inhabiting the richer, warmer climes of the borders. I climb higher to escape the maddening mind-numbing noise. I am not the only one. A group of white doves is spiralling up into the early morning light. A beautiful, peaceful sight above the world's busy awakening, and I sense the soul of an old man released at last from the prison of his lost and confused mind, finding it again – rediscovering his memories. I follow the dwindling flock higher and higher until there is only one dove, large and powerful. The attraction is so great – to find peace at last, away from the hunger that has driven me so far. I fly close to him as he spirals up.

"Don't follow me spirit bird," the voice in my head is gentle, old. "You have a journey to make here. I must leave, you must stay. You can't escape this." The dove, glowing in the fresh morning light, spreads powerful wings and flies straight upwards and disappears, leaving me to glide high above the green of the Pentland Hills.

The pangs of hunger come back, keen and sharp. And with them a fear: have I left it too late? Will I be in time? I speed up – barely taking in the southern hills and plains in the sudden urgency that drives me south. I dread what I will find at the end of my journey, but I must make it.

Then my mind takes a step.

Everything goes blank for a moment, and I flutter down amongst houses, my wings impossibly tired as if I have raced with death itself.

Disorientated and giddy, I see a house that pulls me with its memories. The pretty garden is full of small birds chattering mindlessly, but they scatter as they see me, the blackbird letting off its repetitive warning. I glide round the house looking for some

204

way to see in, and spy a small open window. I am drawn to this with a reluctance that I can't understand. What is so frightening after all this long journey over continents and stormy seas?

I manage to scrabble and squeeze my way through the tiny window and support myself on shaking claws gripping the narrow sill. What strikes me first is the smell: sweet and sickly with a sour tinge to it. Death? No, sick and urine. I look down on the body of a woman. She has been sick and is lying in a pool of urine. A sight so disgusting that I almost fail to see - she is the person I have come for.

She is me.

She is still alive.

Thoughts start coming into my head. In my bird life I had forgotten, now I remember. James - South Downs - paragliding. What for, foolish man? Why leave me like this? There is a sickening blur of memory that I can't face yet. I must go and find him. Now.

My hunger is intense. I will starve soon if I don't find James. I leap off the windowsill, twisting and banging my head in my haste to get going. Every minute counts. I fly high above the rooftops ignoring the bird thoughts that threaten to distract me. I am frantic now. All this driving force that has brought me here is compelling me towards the man I love.

South Downs. Long and wide, green and hilly. There must be people trying to be birds here. I circle high, look down, and there is a group of ungainly fliers, flapping like dishcloths in the morning breeze. I glide down to see if my James is amongst them. Seven of them, flying in various directions and keeping well away from each other. Very sensible under the circumstances - with their lack of control they could easily collide. I pass one after another looking for him. As I fly, my heart begins to beat faster. This is my goal. I must find him.

There at the front of the disparate group, head stretched forward in an ungainly posture as though he is leading a phalanx of migrating geese, is James. As I look at him, it all comes back to me. He loved me. He rescued me, took me in, and I loved him from the first. He will hear me.

"James, you must come home. I need you," I call.

I wing in close so that he can see me. Surely the sight of a raven flying alongside will attract his attention.

He stares straight ahead, eyes fixed on some distant goal of his own.

"James, my love. It's me – I need you to come home." I hear the caw-quack sound that comes from my beak. Can't he hear me? After all this time and journeying it can't be possible that I am unable to speak to him.

"James, James, can you hear me?"

"Cark, cark, caw," is all I can hear coming from me.

This is desperate. I fly in front of him, hoping he will see me. I fly upside down, do a tumble, a somersault, zoom up just missing his face. Nothing.

"James, please, I am dying, you must come home."

He is in a different world. He can't hear me, he can't see me. I fly at him and peck at his hand, he doesn't seem to feel it. My last resort is to fly at his face. I don't want to hurt him so I peck his cheek, carefully avoiding his eyes. No reaction.

I am a spirit bird. To him I am nothing – I don't exist. But I can still try and hear his thoughts. Maybe I can get through to him that way.

Concentrate. Empty my mind to hear his. Something's coming into focus. One word.

"Alice."

Chapter 27

All this way, all this pain, and for what? To discover that my love, my reason for living, is lost to me. Pulled back into his past. His dead love more important than his living one. Not living for much longer.

I can feel myself fading. More spirit than bird, now that the cause of my hunger is gone. But there is something. A question. Do I really want to die because the man I love can't love me? Is he all there is to life? Surely there is more than chasing a man who glides along a sad path, caught in his past. There must be other paths. My life was not worthless before I met him.

Then inside my head, I hear them. The first deep notes of a passacaglia. They pull me with their power. I know that humans can fly in a way, but the man who wrote these notes flew higher than anyone. And the player? I know that player. He puts such deep feeling into his music. The player and the composer are both men who understand unconditional love.

I follow the stream of notes as they develop, leading me an impossible distance in a few bars, and I am outside a chapel in Oxford. The sound of the music is coming out of the arched doorway to the entrance hall of the chapel. I fly in and see the intricate swirling baroque rood screen in front of me. The notes are climbing to the ceiling and I fly up, joining the paintings of angels. There, amongst the glorious notes, I feel almost at home – as though this is what I came all this way for. To rest in Bach's C minor Passacaglia. This noble, glorious, deeply sad creation, telling of love and loss. The repeated line, a bed to lie in, as the growing patterns cover me in ever-changing calico sheets of music.

I don't want him to stop, but I must get him to hear me. I know I will die if he doesn't. I circle down from the high ceiling and spy him in the organ loft, his back turned towards me as he plays, intent upon his music. I see his gently greying hair, a little bald patch developing round his crown. He will soon have the tonsure of a monk, but he is no monk. He loves a woman. He loves me.

The passacaglia is drawing to a close, and I must attract his attention before he goes on to play the fugue. As the final notes gently die away, I fly at a large organ pipe above his head, striking it and making a sudden dull clattering sound amidst all this beautiful music. His head is bowed and his hand is poised to start the fugue. I strike again, more forcefully this time, and he looks up hearing my clatter. I can see that he finds it hard to focus on me. I am a ghostly bird now – a shadow passing above his head. He looks and looks, and then he sees me.

"A bird," he mutters. "Must have left the door open. Fool."

He can see me, at least vaguely. I fly down and perch on the end of the organ console.

"Good God, a raven. A raven in Oxford?" He looks both alarmed and amazed.

"Daniel, Daniel, I need you," I say, just hoping he can hear me in his head through the caw-quack noise I make.

He begins to smile. "This is some kind of joke isn't it. You've brought in a tame bird to wind me up. Is it you Neville? Come on out."

Silence.

"Daniel."

"Who's that? I recognize that voice." Then he suddenly looks sad. "Melissa?"

"Daniel. I need you to come to my house."

"Where are you? You don't need to hide." He peers around the organ loft, trying to see where I could possibly be. Confused, not understanding.

"I am the raven. I have come to find you. I need your help."

He looks at me now. His voice drops to a whisper. "Am I going mad? I've longed to see you all week. Have I turned you into a raven in my head?"

"No, you're not mad. You can hear me. I need you to come to my home. I am dying." The effort in saying this is almost too much for me. I feel myself beginning to fade.

He looks at me, trying to make out what is happening. He shakes his head as if to dismiss all my efforts, and then stares straight ahead. He looks at me, a fading raven, and says in a self-conscious way, "I'm coming."

He whips his jacket off the organ stool, swings his legs round and is running down the stairs, pulling out his mobile phone.

"Where's her number?" he mutters, as he chases through the chapel entrance and across the quad. He presses on my name and listens as he goes. No answer – just answerphone.

"Have I got James?" He belts round a corner of the cloister, nearly colliding with a couple of girl students who laugh as he passes. They can't see me gliding above him. I'm invisible to them.

"Here we are." No reply – just answerphone.

He runs into the car park. Looking round wildly for his car.

He comes to a halt by a black Saab convertible.

"Pull the hood down," I whisper.

He looks puzzled, but gets in, starts the engine, and the hood is coming down as he pulls out of the college car park. Good, I can ride with him. Save my energy.

"East Meon?" He asks himself.

"Yes. Take the A34 south for Winchester." He can hear me. Brilliant.

We make amazing progress out of Oxford. God knows how many speed cameras we speed through. This is Daniel in action mode. The Daniel who rescued me from the library, and from the cold streets of Oxford. Now he is driving with purpose, as though he were a trained racing driver.

We zoom down the busy A34. A slow lorry starts to pull out to overtake an even slower one. I fly in at his open window. He looks shocked and swerves back into the left lane, letting us pass.

He must have been almost asleep, his window open to keep him awake, thank God.

We continue, miraculously unimpeded, down past Newbury. There is less traffic now, and we speed down the outside lane, two black shadows racing to save a life. Time is ticking away. How long have we got? I don't know. I'm still here though – that must mean something.

Winchester. "A31," I whisper. He takes it, and then the small road off it. We must zig-zag our way down narrow roads to my little village.

Daniel pulls up so suddenly that I almost hit the windscreen. There is a tractor in our way, pulling a trailer full of unspeakable muck. He could be going for miles. The road is too narrow for us to pass.

I fly into the back of the driver's cab, and tap on the side window to attract his attention.

He looks round at me. "A bloody raven. Wish I had my gun, I'd shoot it even if it is a bloody protected bird. Kill my lambs it would." He hits out at me angrily catching me off guard, and I hit the side screen of the cab with a painful thud.

Desperately I fly at his face, drawing blood with my sharp beak.

"Fucking hell! Get off!" He is beginning to panic now. A large bird attacking him in a small space. I dodge his attempts to hit me again, and the tractor sways from side to side as we battle. I see a pull-in place coming up on the left of the road, and I make a sudden lunge down at his left hand. He pulls the steering wheel away sharply to avoid my beak, and the tractor turns into the pull-in as he tries to bat me off with his right hand. He brakes hard to avoid hitting a tree, and I leave him cursing and swearing as I fly out to join Daniel as he drives past.

"Thank you," I whisper sarcastically, as we make our way more speedily now. No more tractors, I hope. I don't fancy going through that again.

210

We come into the village at speed. If he doesn't slow down we will be past it before we know it.

"Turn right," I whisper urgently. "And take it slowly."

He does as I ask, and we drive slowly up the high street, cottages to the left and right of us. He stops the car and gets out. He hasn't got a clue where James's house is. I fly ahead, leading him. I am feeling strange now. Disembodied. As though I shouldn't be here any more. My head is spinning as I turn the corner and take him into the front drive of the house. I leave him to find his way in and fly to the bathroom window again. The same stench greets me, but I have to look. Am I still breathing? As I look down from the window light, the bathroom door opens and Daniel sees my body.

"My God," he gasps, and is on his knees in the muck that surrounds me.

I feel myself falling, my final grip on the world weakening as I watch him desperately feeling for my pulse and getting his mobile out. The world is spinning faster and faster now, and I lose all sensation of being in the room. It's getting darker. An oily water surrounds me. It's over my head. I can't breathe. I must get out or I will drown. There is a familiar weight to my movements as I struggle out of the water. I am human. The water streams off my hair as I surface and I can breathe.

Chapter 28

I am walking out of the sea and onto a beach. I have been here before. I have danced on this beach with a child. Now I am alone. The trees stretch from left to right in a great curve in front of me. Behind is the sea with its gentle lapping sound. It has pushed me out and I must go through the wood again to find my way home.

There is something very uncomfortable about the air. Greasy and suffocating. It is difficult to breathe as I make my way unsteadily up the path through the woods to the house. I don't want to go inside this time. This is not home. This is the past, and if I am to survive I must find a future. The 'O' woman is nowhere to be seen as I skirt round the house to the left. This is all unfamiliar. There is a strong smell of vegetation coming from the dark shiny leaves and branches that hem me in. Something warns me that they are poisonous, these dark shiny leaves. I keep close to the house walls, peering in the semi-darkness as I go. I wonder if the house will go on for ever, and whether I will succumb to the poison that I am trying to avoid.

I see it in front of me – light peeping at me, as though at the end of a tunnel. Still the strange oiliness makes it refract in odd ways as though I am only just seeing. Only just there.

I come out of the tunnel, and I find myself at the back of the house. I can see the burnt-out ruins of my old home through the trees. I don't want to go back there either, so I take a gravel path that leads straight past the overgrown garden and down to a lake.

I have been here before too, but seen from this angle, it looks different. I am aware of hills and valleys now – it feels more grown-up, less of a child's garden surrounded by trees. I feel a weight in my hand. The knife. I must give it back. Must never use it again.

On the other side of the lake there is someone watching me. A familiar figure. He was a boy once, now he is a man. Tall and beautiful, he beckons. I loved him once. Now I must give him

213

back his knife.

The edge of the lake is soft to tread on. Water oozes onto my bare feet. At that moment I realise I am completely naked. The scars of feathers are still on my arms – crusty healing scabs. I am thin. Thinner than I've ever been, and I start to feel self-conscious as he stares at me. What does he see? A bony, damaged woman, stiff and awkward. Not the lithe smooth-limbed eye-turner I once was. Life has left its marks all over me.

I round the corner of the lake. Everything is very still, no ripples disturb the surface of the water, no breeze makes the trees rustle, no birds sing. Then I hear it – the sound of a child talking. I can't hear the words, but it sounds plaintive, warm, asking, but sure it is heard.

As I near him the sound stops. I see his eyes. They are not staring at me, they are staring through me to someone behind me. Looking round I can see no-one. Just the lake and the lawns and paths leading down to it.

I go up to him and hold out the knife.

"I think this is yours."

He takes it, and I feel a sense of great sorrow as he turns and walks away from me.

I call after him, but he never turns, or shows any sign that he has heard me. He just walks away into the trees and is lost in their shadows.

I lie down on the soft grass. It bears my weight and I can feel every part of my naked body connecting with the earth. I look up at the blue sky and it begins to turn – slowly at first, then faster and faster until all is a blur. Then darkness.

*

"... found this dead raven on the bathroom floor beside her. Just a ball of feathers and bones. Starved to death, poor thing.

But how it got there…"

Voices are around me as I feel myself being moved on a soft bed. Sheets over me. Smell of hospital. I sleep.

*

Flow my tears, fall from your springs!
Exiled forever, let me mourn;
Where night's black bird her sad infamy sings,
There let me live forlorn.

I hear him sing and play from my bed where I rest, and I feel a sadness that cannot be resolved. I look out of the window at the park and the distant houses beyond, and think of the other one – the one I can never have. I am loved now, but I wonder if I can ever return that love fully. Will a part of me always long for the unattainable?

This man who sings, rescued me. He took me off the streets, and then he saved my life – the only one who could hear me. Now I am safe in his house and I love his music. We share this sound-world in a way that no-one else would understand. He the giver – I the receiver. And yes, I love him, but…

*

Four Years Later - Cotopaxi

Cotopaxi - one of the world's highest active volcanoes. She has worked hard to get here. A driving force that wasn't there before, pushes her on to walk, then run, then fly. Her fear of heights is still there, but it also contains a thrill. That breath-taking drop that was once just the floor, becomes a cliff, and then a mountain. She must fly. Every bone in her body demands this.

The climb up Cotopaxi is long and arduous. They slip and slide up the snow and ice, a whole team is supporting her. She has found numerous sponsors and will raise thousands of pounds with this flight. Daniel has insisted on coming too. He is not all that fit, and struggles. But he is determined to support her in spite of his ageing limbs. He slows them down, and curses himself for doing so, but still they climb and eventually reach the highest part of this great volcano.

Melissa gets strapped into her hang glider. Special extra-warm clothing is put on to stop her freezing during her flight. She is ready to go. Daniel kisses her on the cheek, and stands back, his heart in his mouth, hoping that she will take off and not tumble like a broken raven over the edge of the precipice that she is heading for. There will be no second chance.

She runs down the slope towards the edge, and at the last minute, it seems to him, the air fills her canvas wings and she defies gravity and flies up, catching a thermal, and circles round away from the edge. She turns in flight, and looks at him - is it his imagination or are there tears in her eyes? Much too far away to be sure, but something passes between them, before she turns again and flies away, gradually getting smaller till she becomes a dot in the distance and then disappears entirely.

Acknowledgements

With thanks to my daughter Rose, without whom this story could never have been written; to my daughter-in-law Amy, and in memory of her granny Mary Ash, for giving so much help with search; to Mark Anderson for explaining the cerebellum so to my sister Briony, for her constant inspiration; to Shelley for teaching me such a lot about writing; to Candace r loving my story and encouraging me to stay with rgie Steel for helping me think about transformation; Birkhead, for sending me to the Grand Canyon and ne about ravens; and to my wife Judith, for waking up f tea, and my latest ideas every morning!

s also to Bob Dylan for the inspiration of Mr Tambourine ave always dreamt of dancing beneath a diamond sky daughter Rose. Now we can dance together on the beach hand waving free, in fact with both hands waving free!

About Nick Hooper

Nick Hooper, known as Nicholas Hooper in the film world, is a BAFTA award winning composer, and has written the music for two of the Harry Potter films. Inspired by working so closely with J K Rowling's stories, he turned in 2012 to writing words as well as music. *Above the Void* is the second of three novels, and the third: *The Occasional Gardener*, is due for publication by the end of 2017.